Intermediate
Acupuncture

By Alexander Meng Chao-Lai MD

Translated by Diana Reese-Soltész

Vol. II: Book of Illustrations

With 100 figures

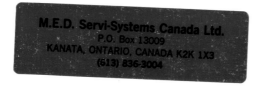

Karl F. Haug Publishers · Heidelberg

CIP-Kurztitelaufnahme der Deutschen Bibliothek

Intermediate acupuncture / transl. by Diana
Reese-Soltész. — Heidelberg : Haug
  Einheitssacht.: Akupunktur für mässig
  Fortgeschrittene ⟨engl.⟩
  Bd. 2 zu: Bischko, Johannes: An introduction
  to acupuncture
  ISBN 3-7760-0888-1
NE: Reese-Soltész, Diana [Übers.]; EST

(Book of illustrations). By Alexander Meng
Chao-Lai. — 1986.
NE: Meng, Alexander Chao-Lai [Mitverf.]

Herstellerische Betreuung: Axel Treiber

Publisher's number 8605
ISBN 3-7760-0888-1
This book is also available in a German and in a Portuguese edition.
Typeset by Filmsatz Unger, 6940 Weinheim, Federal Republic of Germany
Printed by Pilger-Druckerei, 6720 Speyer, Federal Republic of Germany

Table of Contents

Introduction

When the manuscript of the original German-language version of this book was finished, we were faced with a big problem. Time after time, my staff at the institute and I heard from seminar participants the demand for more slides, more pictures, more tables, etc. That demand is very hard to fulfill. The acupuncture needles are so thin that they are only visible in close-ups, which in turn cannot, of course, show any other loci except for the one in question to facilitate orientation. The result is a photograph of skin with a needle stuck into it and nothing else.

Anatomic drawings alone, on the other hand, do not show skin creases, reference points of nerves and vessels, or other relevant spaces to serve orientation.

Having little talent for drawing myself, I am very grateful to my collaborator, *Meng,* for having put together a complete book of figures to complement my textbook. We agreed that it would be best not to draw large figures, but rather, a separate one for each control loop, and that being able to use the textbook and the illustrations at the same time would make it easier for the reader to understand and memorize.

Some control loops required frontal and dorsal, and at times, even lateral views. The numbers of the corresponding figures are mentioned repeatedly in the textbook.

I must, however, emphasize one thing. No matter how good and exact a visual aid may be, it can never substitute one's own sense of touch and exact knowledge of the individual points' locations. As mentioned in the textbook, point detectors may be quite useful for finding points on certain areas of the body (e. g. abdomen, back).

We would like to hear from you, the reader, especially whether or not the option we have chosen really is useful, in daily practice as well.

That is how **Intermediate Acupuncture** came to be two books, which, however, form an inseparable unit. Our thanks go to our publisher for his understanding and fine layout, and to our translator, *Diana Reese-Soltész.* To you, the reader, go our best wishes and sincerest hopes that our combined efforts will be to your benefit.

Vienna, April 1986

Prof. *J. Bischko,* M. D.   *A. Meng Chao-Lai,* M. D.

7

Foreword

It was a great honor for me to draw the illustrations to the textbook, **Intermediate Acupuncture** by my revered teacher, *Bischko*.

Some pertinent problems in acupuncture are revealed thereby: first of all, the diverging data on points' locations, and secondly, the depth of needle insertion.

The points I have drawn conform exclusively to *Bischko's* descriptions of their locations in the 2nd edition of **An Introduction to Acupuncture** and the **Intermediate Acupuncture** Textbook. The data pertaining to the control loops (feedback mechanisms) are based on *Bischko's* over 30 years of clinical experience on well over ten-thousand patients. These data (point locations, indications) have also been confirmed by the over thousand physicians who have studied at the institute (myself, as so-called representative of Chinese acupuncture at the Boltzmann Institute included), and the results achieved therewith on our patients. The diverging numeration of the meridian points (e.g. Meridian of the Bladder) and the discrepancies in point locations in different acupuncture books are in part due to historical reasons. The 361 meridian points evolved in the course of approx. over 3,000 years of development. Several times within that time span, great scholars in China made extensive changes in the acupuncture points' associations with a respective meridian, location, indication, and names. The last − for the time being − extensive re-classification of acupuncture terminology (resembling the anatomic terminology of customary Occidental medicine) was done in the last approx. 35 years in the People's Republic of China. International nomenclature is contained herein.

Decisive for obtaining desired results is the locus where the needle is placed, and not its number. For example, with the point Lung 11, its location being on the ulnar corner of the cuticle of the thumb, efficacious acupuncture analgesia for tonsillectomy may be done. That is, however, not the case when the location described more recently by Chinese sources, i. e. radial to the cuticle of the thumb is used *(Bischko)*. Another example is LI 4, recent Chinese sources describing its location as being radial to the second metacarpal bone, exactly in the middle, whereas *Bischko* describes it as being in the proximal angle between the first and second metacarpal bones. *Bischko's* location is more suitable for superficial needling; the Chinese for deep needling (similarly to the point G 30 among others).

And now to the second problem: Is superficial needling as has been practiced for years by *Bischko,* all his teachers, and pupils, still valid when we now know that our Chinese colleagues insert the needles much deeper? I discussed the topic at great length with Chinese colleagues during my studies at the Academy of Traditional Chinese Medicine in Shanghai in 1979.

My personal opinion is that superficial needling produces good results in about 80% of our acupuncture patients. In the outpatient service of the Ludwig Boltzmann Acupuncture Institute, about 10,000 individual treatments are given each year. Of course, we also use the method of deeper needle insertion for cases of paralysis, therapy-resistance, disorders requiring special types of acupuncture procedures, acupuncture analgesia, etc. However, the majority of patients we encounter in our outpatient service and in our own offices have chronic disorders. They are very sensitive individuals, their disorders usually having psychological components. Such patients are grateful not to be irritated too strongly with the needle, and the majority respond to even superficial needling (depth of insertion: 1 – 2 mm) with plainly visible local reddening around the inserted needle. Most of the patients report feeling a sensation of warmth, tingling ... the so-called Deqi, or needle, sensation. The same sensation is also demanded of deep needling with steel needles.

Is the technique of superficial needling known of in traditional Chinese medicine? Certainly. Therein, the gentle, weak stimulus is considered to be a *tonifying* stimulus, and the strong, intense stimulus, a *sedating* one. Any acute, recent disorder (so-called Yang states) must be approached with the sedating technique (deeper needle insertion, more manipulation of the needle, more intense perception of the stimulus on the part of the patient). On the other hand, any disorder of long-standing, as well as psychosomatic disorders (Yin states), require tonification (weaker stimulus, superficial needle insertion). The so-called Yin states comprise about 80% of Central European acupuncture patients.

Conversely, in the People's Republic of China, more than 90% of acupuncture patients have Yang conditions (acute, only recent disorders). That explains the completely different point combinations, needling technique, and success rates there. A not unsubstantial role is also played by the patient's mentality and acupuncture's position in Chinese medical care as a whole.

In summarizing, I advise all of you to always needle superficially the loci presented herein for the indications in the textbook of **Intermediate Acupuncture** with short gold and silver needles. Only in the event that still no reaction has been achieved after 4 – 10 treatments, should the technique of intensified stimulation: deeper insertion of steel needles, be used.

All the figures have been carefully checked. Should you nevertheless find errors therein, please let us know. My heartiest thanks go to all my colleagues, who have given me such valuable incentives, as well as to the publishers.

Vienna, April 1986   *Chao-Lai Alexander Meng,* M. D.

Index of the Figures

14

Part I

**The 100 Illustrations of the Control Loops,
the Points Thereof, and Descriptions of the Locations
of the Cited Points**

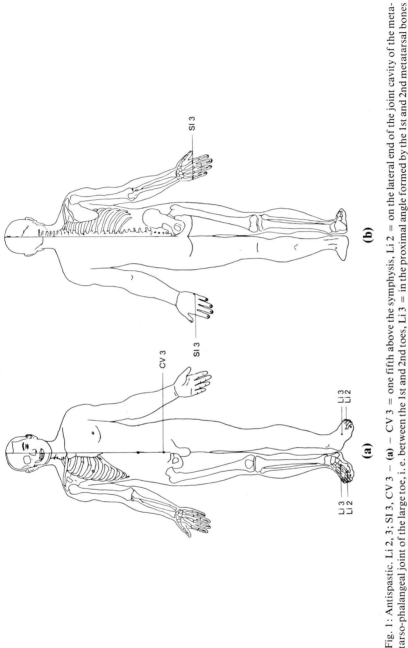

(a)

(b)

Fig. 1: Antispastic. Li 2, 3; SI 3, CV 3 – **(a)** – CV 3 = one fifth above the symphysis, Li 2 = on the lateral end of the joint cavity of the metatarso-phalangeal joint of the large toe, i.e. between the 1st and 2nd toes, Li 3 = in the proximal angle formed by the 1st and 2nd metatarsal bones – **(b)** – SI 3 = on the lateral end of the skin crease behind (proximal to) the metacarpo-phalangeal joint of the small finger which is formed when the hand is closed in a fist.

21

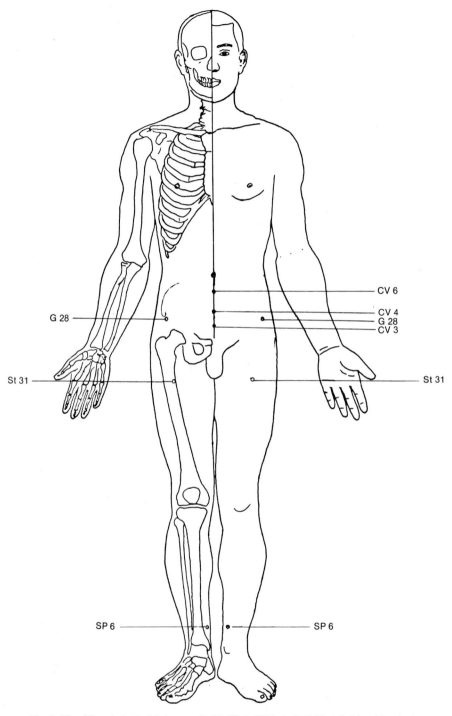

CV 6

CV 4
G 28
CV 3

G 28

St 31

St 31

SP 6

SP 6

Fig. 2: Blood Supply in the Mesentery. St 31, SP 6, CV 3, 4, 6; G 28 − St 31 = identical to
Li 12, SP 6 = point of intersection; approx. 4 fingerbreadths above the internal malleolus,
CV 3 = one fifth above the symphysis, CV 4 = two fifths above the symphysis, CV 6 = 2
fingerbreadths below the navel, G 28 = on the anterior superior iliac spine.

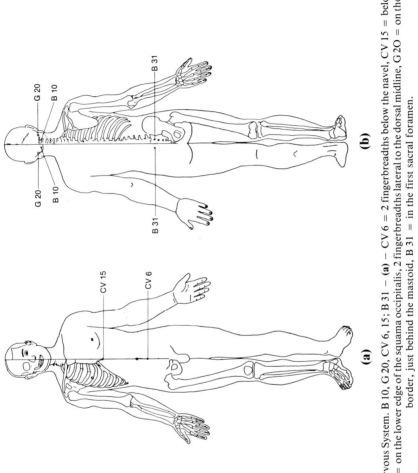

Fig. 3: Autonomic Nervous System. B 10, G 20, CV 6, 15; B 31 – **(a)** – CV 6 = 2 fingerbreadths below the navel, CV 15 = below the tip of the xiphoid – **(b)** – B 10 = on the lower edge of the squama occipitalis, 2 fingerbreadths lateral to the dorsal midline, G 2O = on the lower occipital border, just behind the mastoid, B 31 = in the first sacral foramen.

23

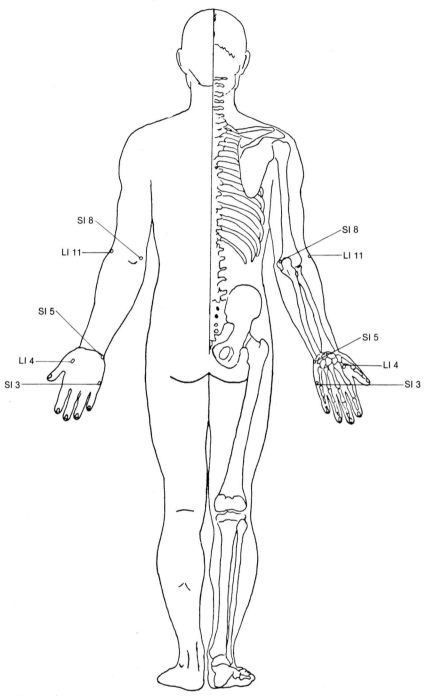

Fig. 4: Mucous Membrane. LI 4, 11; SI 3, 5, 8 − LI 4 = in the proximal angle between the 1st and 2nd metacarpal bones, LI 11 = on the lateral end of the crease of the elbow, SI 3 = on the lateral end of the skin crease proximal to the metacarpophalangeal joint of the small finger which is formed when the hand is closed in a first, SI 5 = distal to the processus styloideus ulnae, SI 8 = on the lower part of the edge of the olecranon.

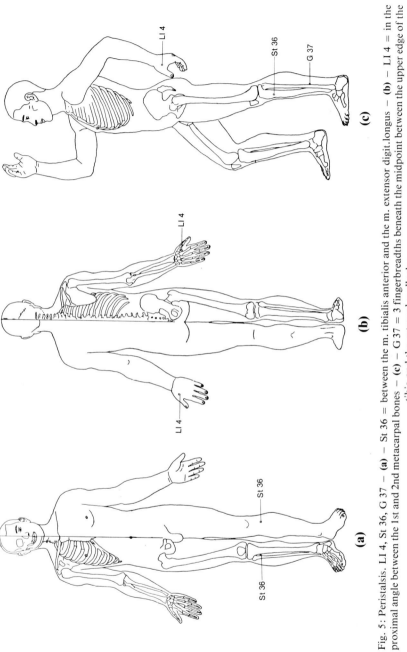

(a)

(b)

(c)

Fig. 5: Peristalsis. LI 4, St 36, G 37 — **(a)** — St 36 = between the m. tibialis anterior and the m. extensor digit.longus — **(b)** — LI 4 = in the proximal angle between the 1st and 2nd metacarpal bones — **(c)** — G 37 = 3 fingerbreadths beneath the midpoint between the upper edge of the tibia and the external malleolus.

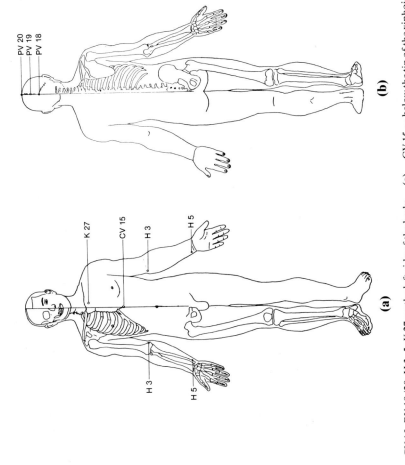

Fig. 6: Psyche. CV 15, PV 19/20, H 3, 5; K 27 on the left side of the body – **(a)** – CV 15 = below the tip of the xiphoid, H 3 = on the medial end of the crease of the elbow, H 5 = on the level of the ulnar apophysis, K 27 = on the edge of the sternum, on the lower part of the sternoclavicular joint – **(b)** – PV 19 = on the point of intersection of the lambdoid and sagittal sutures, PV 20 = on the highest point of the crown.

26

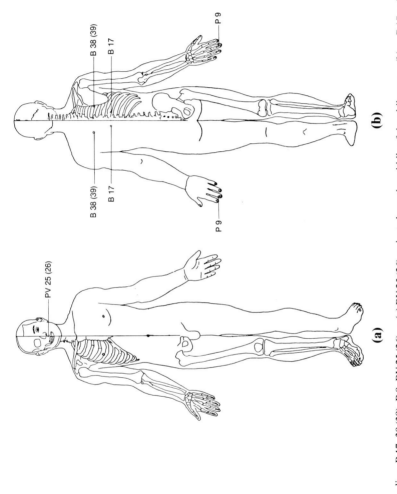

(a)

(b)

Fig. 7: Bleeding. B 17, 38 (39), P 9, PV 25 (26) – **(a)** PV 25 (26) = just above the middle of the philtrum – **(b)** – B 17 = between the 7th and 8th thoracic vertebrae, B 38 (39) = on the point of intersection of the scapula and the upper edge of the fourth rib, P 9 = 2 mm medial and proximal to the corner of the cuticle of the middle finger (thumb side).

27

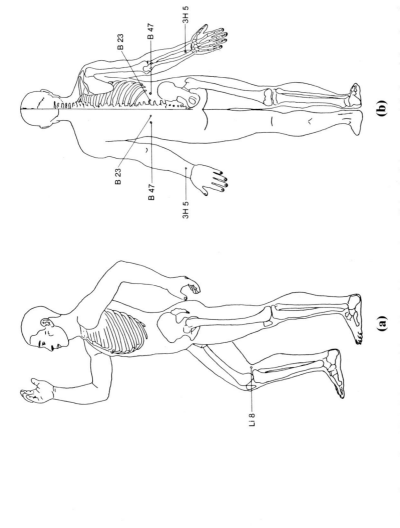

(a)

(b)

Fig. 8: Inflammation. 3H 5, B 23, 47; Li 8 – **(a)** – Li 8 = on the medial end of the crease of the knee joint when the knee is maximally bent – **(b)** – 3H 5 = just 3 fingerbreadths above the capitulum ulnae, B 23 = between the 2nd and 3rd lumbar vertebrae, B 47 = 1 fingerbreadth above the iliac crest and 4 fingerbreadths lateral to the dorsal midline.

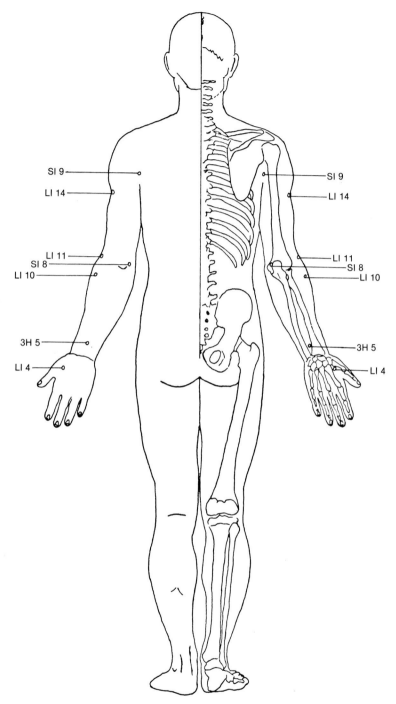

Fig. 9: Arm. Ll 4, 10, 11, 14; SI 8, 9; 3H 5 – LI 4 = in the proximal angle between the 1st and 2nd metacarpal bones, LI 10 = 2 fingerbreadths distal to LI 11, LI 11 = on the lateral end of the crease of the elbow, LI 14 = on the lowest point of attachment of the deltoid muscle on the upper arm, SI 8 = on the lower portion of the edge of the olecranon, SI 9 = 2 fingerbreadths above the dorsal end of the axillar fold, 3H 5 = just 3 fingerbreadths above the capitulum ulnae.

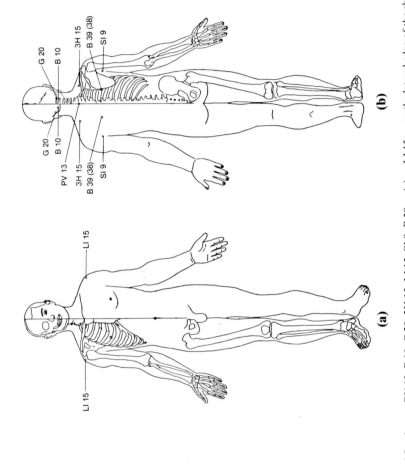

Fig. 10: Cervical Syndrome. PV 13, B 10, G 20, 3H 15, LI 15, SI 9, B 39 – **(a)** – LI 15 = on the lateral edge of the shoulder in the indentation below the acromion – **(b)** – PV 13 = on C 7, B 10 = on the lower edge of the squama occipitalis, 2 fingerbreadths lateral to the dorsal midline, G 20 = on the lower occipital border, just behind the mastoid, 3H 15 = on the upper edge of the trapezius in the middle of the shoulder, LI 15 = on the lateral edge of the shoulder in the indentation below the acromion, SI 9 = 2 fingerbreadths above the dorsal end of the axillary fold, B 39 = on the point of intersection of the scapula and the upper edge of the 4th rib.

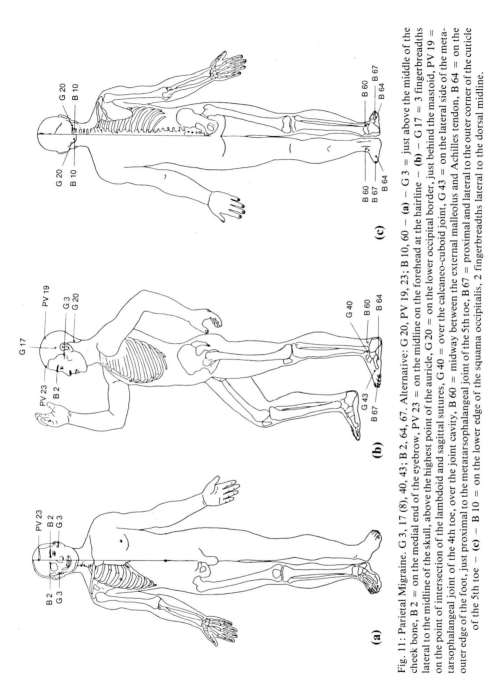

Fig. 11: Parietal Migraine. G 3, 17 (8), 40, 43; B 2, 64, 67. Alternative: G 20, PV 19, 23; B 10, 60 − **(a)** − G 3 = just above the middle of the cheek bone, B 2 = on the medial end of the eyebrow, PV 23 = on the midline on the forehead at the hairline − **(b)** − G 17 = 3 fingerbreadths lateral to the midline of the skull, above the highest point of the auricle, G 20 = on the lower occipital border, just behind the mastoid, PV 19 = on the point of intersection of the lambdoid and sagittal sutures, G 40 = over the calcaneo-cuboid joint, G 43 = on the lateral side of the metatarsophalangeal joint of the 4th toe, over the joint cavity, B 60 = midway between the external malleolus and Achilles tendon, B 64 = on the outer edge of the foot, just proximal to the metatarsophalangeal joint of the 5th toe, B 67 = proximal and lateral to the outer corner of the cuticle of the 5th toe − **(c)** − B 10 = on the lower edge of the squama occipitalis, 2 fingerbreadths lateral to the dorsal midline.

31

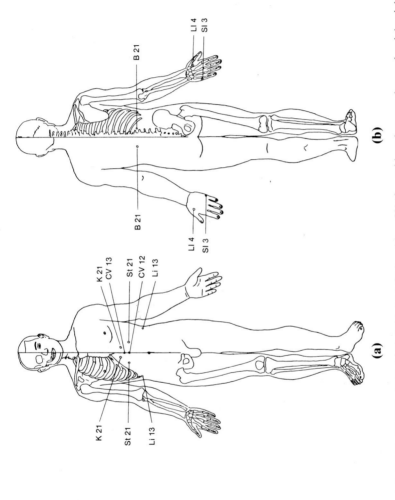

(a)

(b)

Fig. 12: Stomach. CV 12, 13; K 21, St 21, Li 13, B 21, Li 4, SI 3 — **(a)** — CV 12 = midway between the navel and the xiphoid, CV 13 = three eighths below the tip of the xiphoid, K 21 = on the tip of the angle between the 6th and 7th costal cartilage on the level of the 6th intercostal space, St 21 = in the angle of the 8th intercostal space, often 1 fingerbreadth medial thereto, Li 13 = on the free end of the 11th rib. — **(b)** — B 21 = between the 12th thoracic and 1st lumbar vertebrae, Li 4 = in the proximal angle between the 1st and 2nd metacarpal bones, SI 3 = on the lateral end of the skin fold behind (proximal to) the metacarpophalangeal joint of the small finger, when the hand is closed in a fist.

32

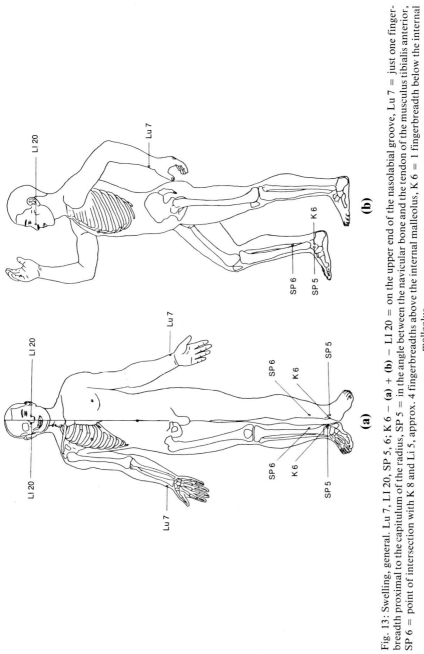

(b)

(a)

Fig. 13: Swelling, general. Lu 7, Ll 20, SP 5, 6; K 6 – **(a)** + **(b)** – Ll 20 = on the upper end of the nasolabial groove, Lu 7 = just one finger-breadth proximal to the capitulum of the radius, SP 5 = in the angle between the navicular bone and the tendon of the musculus tibialis anterior, SP 6 = point of intersection with K 8 and Li 5, approx. 4 fingerbreadths above the internal malleolus, K 6 = 1 fingerbreadth below the internal malleolus.

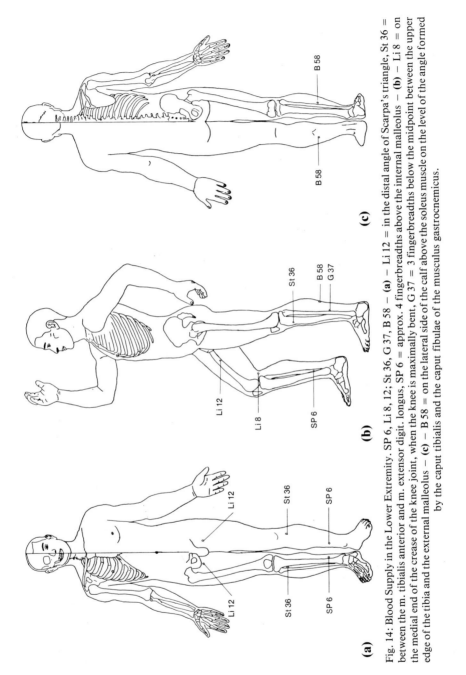

(a)

Li 12

St 36

SP 6

Li 12

St 36

SP 6

(b)

Li 12

Li 8

SP 6

St 36

B 58
G 37

(c)

B 58

B 58

Fig. 14: Blood Supply in the Lower Extremity. SP 6, Li 8, 12; St 36, G 37, B 58 – **(a)** – Li 12 = in the distal angle of Scarpa's triangle, St 36 = between the m. tibialis anterior and m. extensor digit. longus, SP 6 = approx. 4 fingerbreadths above the internal malleolus – **(b)** – Li 8 = on the medial end of the crease of the knee joint, when the knee is maximally bent, G 37 = 3 fingerbreadths below the midpoint between the upper edge of the tibia and the external malleolus – **(c)** – B 58 = on the lateral side of the calf above the soleus muscle on the level of the angle formed by the caput tibialis and the caput fibulae of the musculus gastrocnemicus.

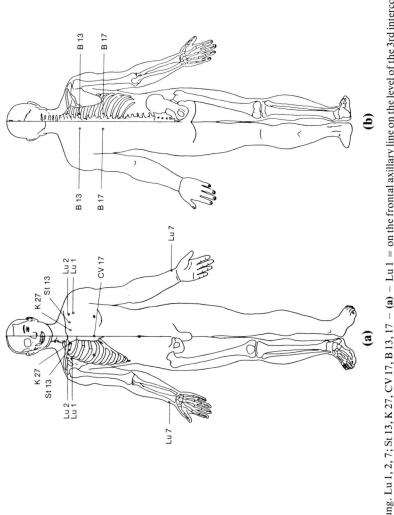

(b)

(a)

Fig. 15: Lung. Lu 1, 2, 7; St 13, K 27, CV 17, B 13, 17 – **(a)** – Lu 1 = on the frontal axillary line on the level of the 3rd intercostal space, Lu 2 = same as Lu 1, but in the 2nd intercostal space, Lu 7 = just 1 fingerbreadth proximal to the capitulum of the radius, St 13 = on the lower edge of the clavicle, approx. in the middle, K 27 = on the edge of the sternum, on the lower part of the sternoclavicular joint, CV 17 = in the middle of the sternum on the level of the 6th intercostal space – **(b)** – B 13 = between the 3rd and 4th thoracic vertebrae, B 17 = between the 7th and 8th thoracic vertebrae.

35

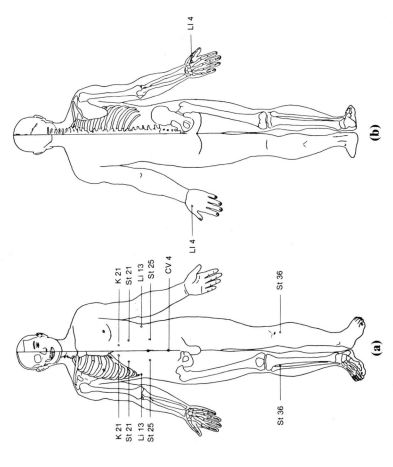

K 21
St 21
Li 13
St 25
CV 4

St 36

Li 4

(a)

Li 4

Li 4

St 36

(b)

Fig. 16: Large Intestine. Li 4, St 21, 25, 36; Li 13, K 21, CV 4 – **(a)** – K 21 = on the tip of the angle between the 6th and 7th costal cartilage, St 21 = in the angle of the 8th intercostal space, often 1 fingerbreadth medial thereto, St 25 = approx. 2 fingerbreadths lateral to the navel, or midway between the navel and the anterior superior iliac crest, Li 13 = on the free end of the 11th rib, CV 4 = two fifths above the symphysis, St 36 = between the m. tibialis anterior and m. extensor digit. longus – **(b)** – Li 4 = in the proximal angle between the 1st and 2nd metacarpal bones.

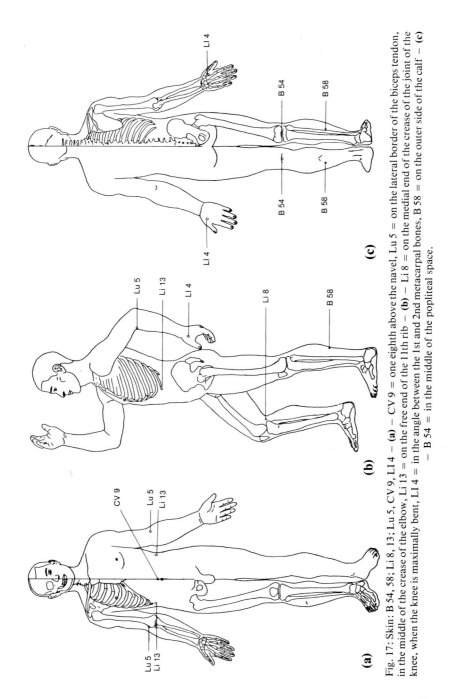

(a)

(b)

(c)

Fig. 17: Skin: B 54, 58; Li 8, 13; Lu 5, 13; Lu 5, Li 8, 13; Lu 5, CV 9, LI 4 – **(a)** – CV 9 = one eighth above the navel, Lu 5 = on the lateral border of the biceps tendon, in the middle of the crease of the elbow, Li 13 = on the free end of the 11th rib – **(b)** – Li 8 = on the medial end of the crease of the joint of the knee, when the knee is maximally bent, LI 4 = in the angle between the 1st and 2nd metacarpal bones, B 58 = on the outer side of the calf – **(c)** – B 54 = in the middle of the popliteal space.

37

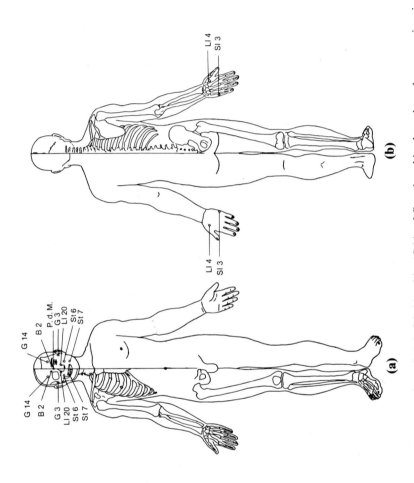

(a)

G 14

B 2

P. d. M.

G 3

LI 20

St 6

St 7

G 14

B 2

G 3

LI 20

St 6

St 7

LI 4

SI 3

(b)

LI 4

SI 3

Fig. 18: Sinuses. LI 4, 20; B 2, SI 3, P. d. M., St 6, 7; G 3, 14 – **(a)** – G 14 = 2 fingerbreadths above the eyebrow on an imaginary perpendicular line through the middle of the pupil, B 2 = on the medial end of the eyebrow, P. d. M., Point de Merveille = in the middle of the root of the nose, G 3 = just above the middle of the cheek bone, LI 20 = on the upper end of the nasolabial groove, St 6 = on an imaginary perpendicular line through the middle of the pupil on the level of the nostril, St 7 = on the point of intersection of an imaginary perpendicular line through the middle of the pupil and the corner of the mouth – **(b)** – LI 4 = in the proximal angle between the 1st and 2nd metacarpal bones, SI 3 = on the lateral end of the skin fold behind (proximal to) the metacarpophalangeal joint of the small finger when the hand is closed in a fist.

38

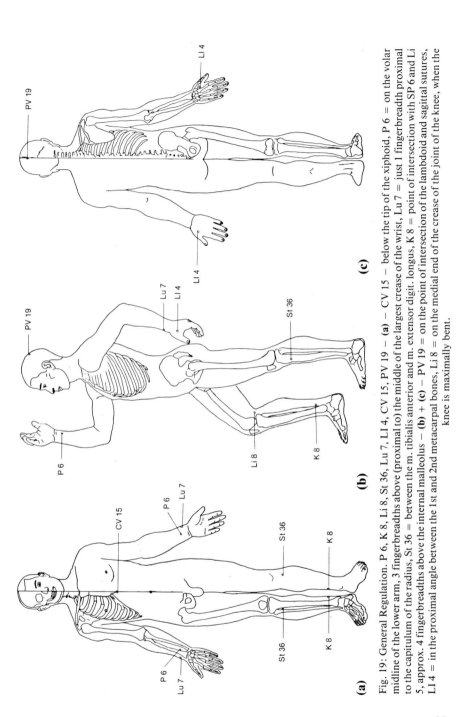

Fig. 19: General Regulation. P 6, K 8, Li 8, St 36, Lu 7, LI 4, CV 15, PV 19 – **(a)** – CV 15 – below the tip of the xiphoid, P 6 = on the volar midline of the lower arm, 3 fingerbreadths above (proximal to) the middle of the largest crease of the wrist, Lu 7 = just 1 fingerbreadth proximal to the capitulum of the radius, St 36 = between the m. tibialis anterior and m. extensor digit. longus, K 8 = point of intersection with SP 6 and Li 5, approx. 4 fingerbreadths above the internal malleolus – **(b)** + **(c)** – PV 19 = on the point of intersection of the lambdoid and sagittal sutures, LI 4 = in the proximal angle between the 1st and 2nd metacarpal bones, Li 8 = on the medial end of the crease of the joint of the knee, when the knee is maximally bent.

39

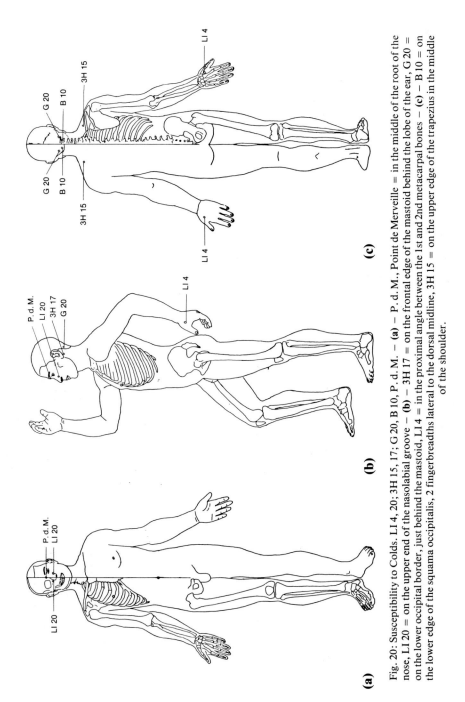

Fig. 20: Susceptibility to Colds. LI 4, 20; 3H 15, 17; G 20, B 10, P. d. M. – (a) – P. d. M., Point de Merveille = in the middle of the root of the nose, LI 20 = on the upper end of the nasolabial groove – (b) – 3H 17 = on the frontal edge of the mastoid behind the lobe of the ear, G 20 = on the lower occipital border, just behind the mastoid, LI 4 = in the proximal angle between the 1st and 2nd metacarpal bones – (c) – B 10 = on the lower edge of the squama occipitalis, 2 fingerbreadths lateral to the dorsal midline, 3H 15 = on the upper edge of the trapezius in the middle of the shoulder.

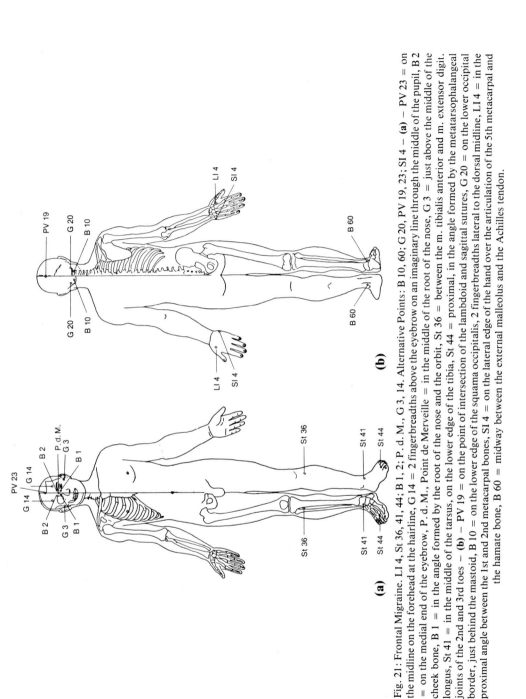

Fig. 21: Frontal Migraine. LI 4, St 36, 41, 44; B 1, 2; P. d. M., G 3, 14. Alternative Points: B 10, 60; G 20, PV 19, 23; SI 4 – (a) – PV 23 = on the midline on the forehead at the hairline, G 14 = 2 fingerbreadths above the eyebrow on an imaginary line through the middle of the pupil, B 2 = on the medial end of the eyebrow, P. d. M., Point de Merveille = in the middle of the root of the nose, G 3 = just above the middle of the cheek bone, B 1 = in the angle formed by the root of the nose and the orbit, St 36 = between the m. tibialis anterior and m. extensor digit. longus, St 41 = in the middle of the tarsus, on the lower edge of the tibia, St 44 = proximal, in the angle formed by the metatarsophalangeal joints of the 2nd and 3rd toes – (b) – PV 19 = on the point of intersection of the lambdoid and sagittal sutures, G 20 = on the lower occipital border, just behind the mastoid, B 10 = on the lower edge of the squama occipitalis, 2 fingerbreadths lateral to the dorsal midline, LI 4 = in the proximal angle between the 1st and 2nd metacarpal bones, SI 4 = on the lateral edge of the hand over the articulation of the 5th metacarpal and the hamate bone, B 60 = midway between the external malleolus and the Achilles tendon.

41

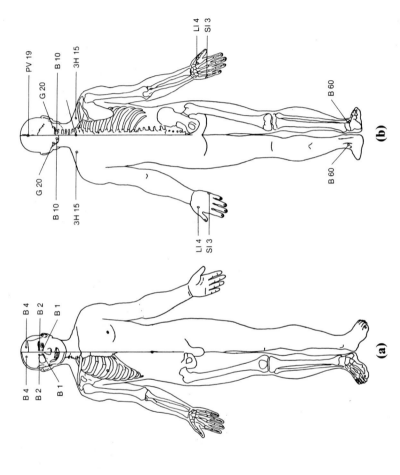

Fig. 22: Cervical Migraine. B 1, 2, 4, 10; G 20, PV 13, 19. Alternative Points: B 60, LI 4, SI 3, 3H 15 — **(a)** — B 4 = approx. 2 fingerbreadths lateral to the midline, approx. 2 fingerbreadths above the hairline, B 2 = on the medial end of the eyebrow, B 1 = in the angle formed by the root of the nose and the orbit — **(b)** — PV 19 = on the point of intersection of the lambdoid and sagittal sutures, G 20 = on the lower occipital border, just behind the mastoid, B 10 = on the lower edge of the squama occipitalis, 2 fingerbreadths lateral to the dorsal midline, PV 13 = on C 7, 3H 15 = on the upper edge of the trapezius in the middle of the shoulder, LI 4 = in the proximal angle between the 1st and 2nd metacarpal bones, SI 3 = on the lateral end of the skin fold behind (proximal to) the metacarpophalangeal joint of the small finger when the hand is closed in a fist, B 60 = midway between the external malleolus and the Achilles tendon.

42

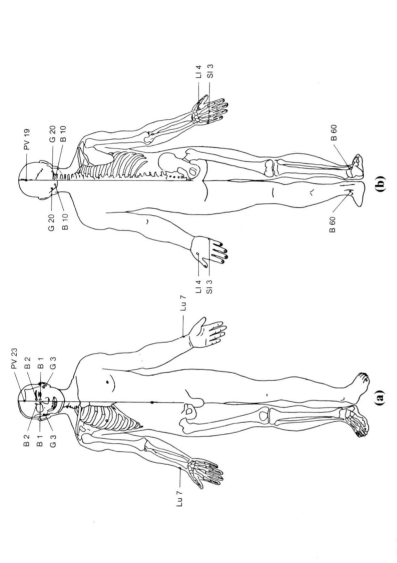

Fig. 23: Cephalaea, general. PV 19, 23; B 1, 2, 10; G 3, 20. Alternative Points: B 60, LI 4, SI 3, Lu 7 – **(a)** – PV 23 = on the midline on the forehead at the hairline, B 2 = on the medial end of the eyebrow, B 1 = in the angle formed by the root of the nose and the orbit, G 3 = just above the middle of the cheek bone, Lu 7 = just 1 fingerbreadth above the capitulum of the radius – **(b)** – PV 19 = on the point of intersection of the lambdoid and sagittal sutures, G 20 = on the lower occipital border, just behind the mastoid, B 10 = on the lower edge of the squama occipitalis, 2 fingerbreadths lateral to the dorsal midline, LI 4 = in the proximal angle between the 1st and 2nd metacarpal bones, SI 3 = on the lateral end of the skin fold behind (proximal to) the metacarpophalangeal joint of the small finger, when the hand is closed in a fist, B 60 = midway between the external malleolus and the Achilles tendon.

43

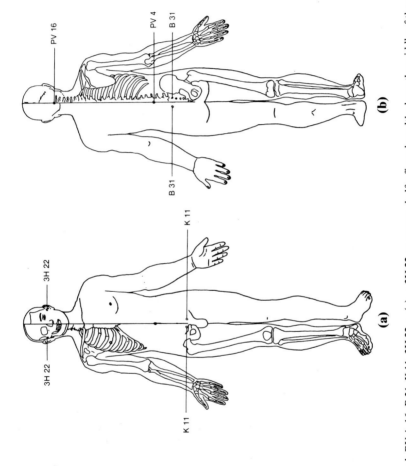

(a)

(b)

Fig. 24: Hormonal. PV 4, 16; B 31, K 11, 3H 22 – **(a)** – 3H 22 = approx. half a fingerbreadth above the middle of the cheek bone, K 11 = on the upper edge of the pubis, approx. 2 (or 1) fingerbreadths lateral to the midline – **(b)** – PV 16 = on the midline, on the lower occipital border, PV 4 = on L 3, B 31 = in the 1st sacral foramen.

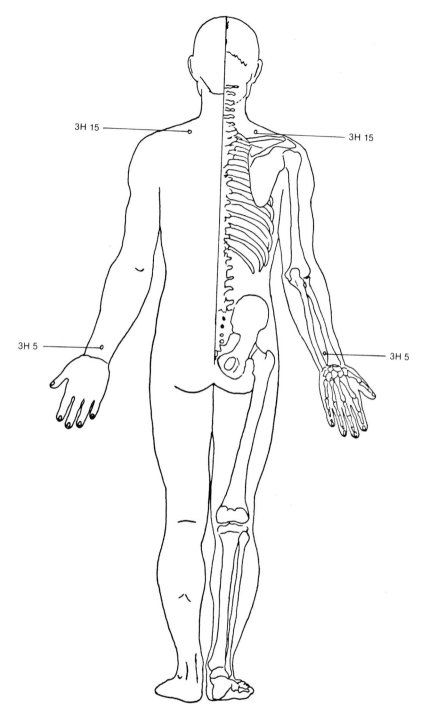

3H 15

3H 15

3H 5

3H 5

Fig. 25: Sensitivity to Weather. 3H 15, 3H 5 – 3H 15 = on the upper edge of the trapezius in the middle of the shoulder, 3H 5 = just 3 fingerbreadths above the capitulum ulnae.

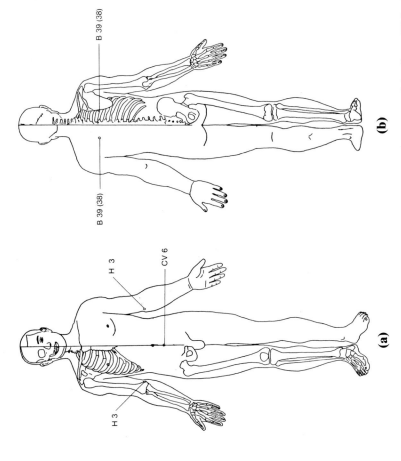

(a)

(b)

Fig. 26: Depressive State. H 3, CV 6, perhaps B 39 – **(a)** – H 3 = on the medial end of the crease of the elbow, CV 6 = 2 fingerbreadths below the navel – **(b)** – B 39 = on the point of intersection of the scapula and the upper edge of the 4th rib.

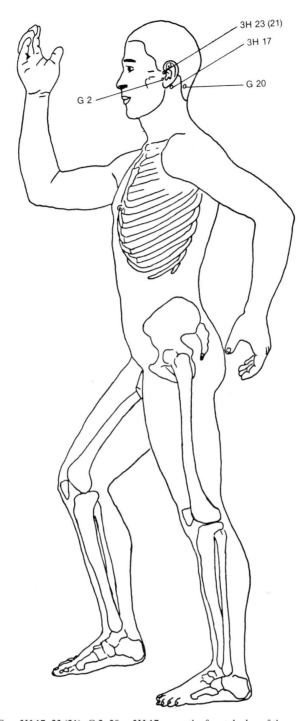

Fig. 27: Ear. 3H 17, 23 (21); G 2, 20 − 3H 17 = on the frontal edge of the mastoid behind the lobe of the ear, 3H 23 = in the indentation between the tragus and the upper point of attachment of the auricle, G 20 = on the lower occipital border, just behind the mastoid, G 2 = on the level of the incisura intertragica inferior.

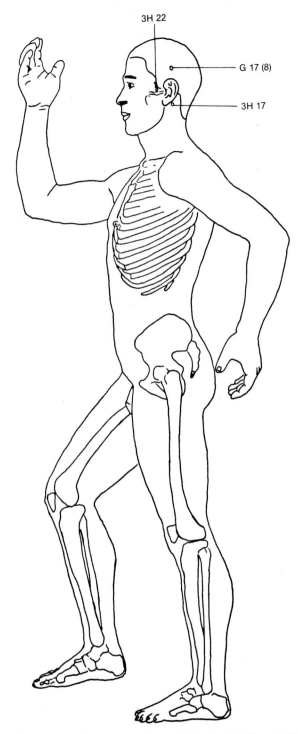

Fig. 28: Blood Supply in the Head, Parietal Part. 3H 17, 22; G 17 (8) − 3 H 22 = approx. half a fingerbreadth above the middle of the cheek bone, G 17 = 3 fingerbreadths lateral to the midline of the skull above the highest point of the auricle, 3H 17 = on the frontal edge of the mastoid, behind the lobe of the ear.

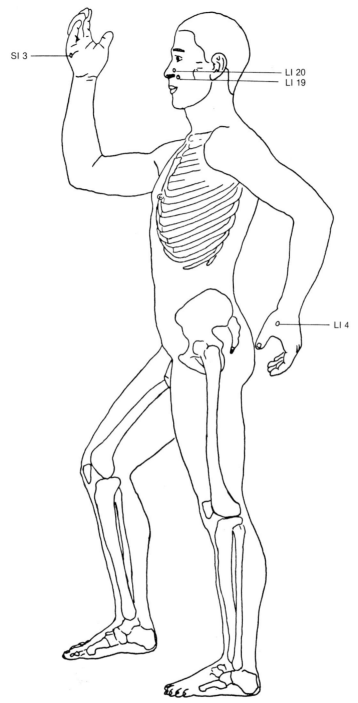

Fig. 29: Nasal Mucous Membrane. LI 4, 19, 20; SI 3 − SI 3 = on the lateral end of the skin fold behind (proximal to) the metacarpophalangeal joint of the small finger, when the hand is closed in a fist, LI 20 = on the upper end of the nasolabial groove, LI 19 = in the nasolabial groove on the level of the nostrils, LI 4 = in the proximal angle between the 1st and 2nd metacarpal bones.

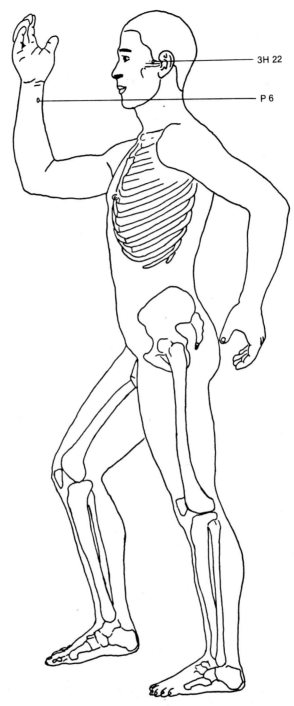

Fig. 30: Nasal Blood Supply. P 6, 3H 22 − P 6 = on the volar midline of the lower arm, approximately 3 fingerbreadths above the largest crease of the wrist, 3H 22 = approx. half a fingerbreadth above the middle of the cheek bone.

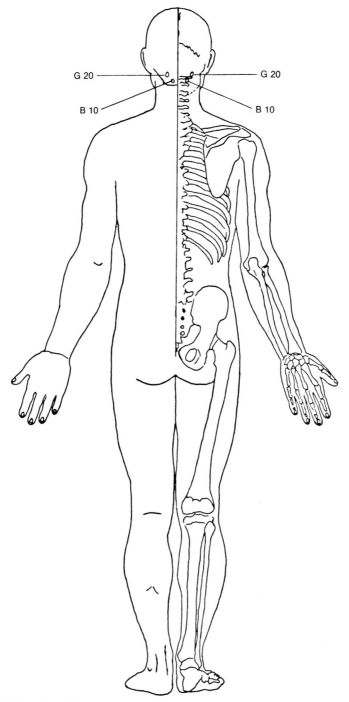

Fig. 31: Nose, Opposition. B 10 and/or G 20 − B 10 = on the lower edge of the squama occipitalis, 2 fingerbreadths lateral to the dorsal midline, G 20 = on the lower occipital border, just behind the mastoid.

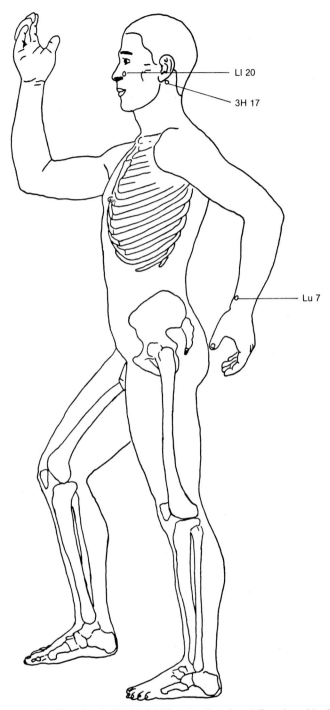

Fig. 32: Nose, Swelling. Lu 7, 3H 17, LI 20 — Lu 7 = just 1 fingerbreadth above the capitulum of the radius, 3H 17 = on the frontal edge of the mastoid, behind the lobe of the ear, LI 20 = on the upper end of the nasolabial groove.

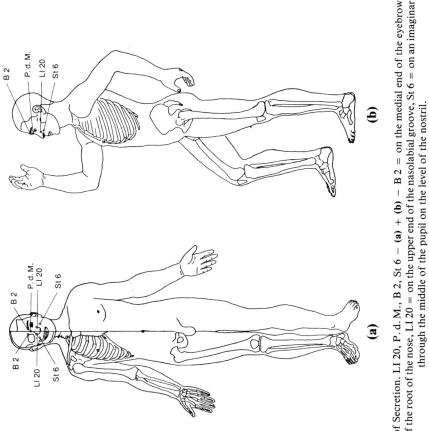

(b)

(a)

Fig. 33: Nose, Promotion of Secretion. LI 20, P. d. M., B 2, St 6 – **(a)** + **(b)** – B 2 = on the medial end of the eyebrow, P. d. M., Point de Merveille = in the middle of the root of the nose, LI 20 = on the upper end of the nasolabial groove, St 6 = on an imaginary perpendicular line through the middle of the pupil on the level of the nostril.

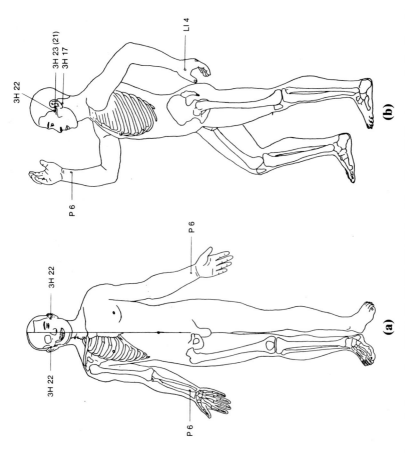

Fig. 34: Trigeminal Nerve – Inflammation. 3H 17, 22, 23 (21); LI4, P 6 – (a) + (b) – 3H 22 = approx. half a fingerbreadth above the middle of the cheek bone, P 6 = on the volar midline of the lower arm, approx. 3 fingerbreadths above the largest crease of the wrist, 3H 23 (21) = in the indentation between the tragus and point of attachment of the auricle, 3H 17 = on the frontal edge of the mastoid, behind the lobe of the ear, LI 4 = in the proximal angle between the 1st and 2nd metacarpal bones.

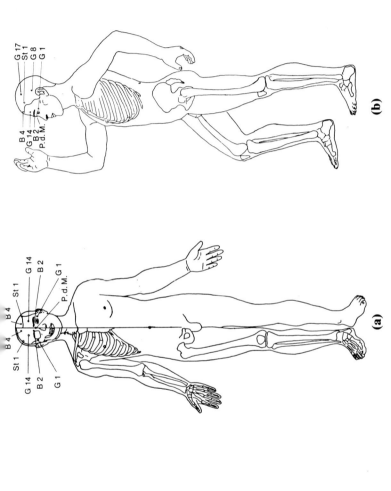

(a)

(b)

Fig. 35: Trigeminal Nerve, 1st Branch. G 1, 8, 14, 17; P. d. M., B 2, 4; St 1 – **(a)** – B 4 = approx. 2 fingerbreadths lateral to the midline, about 2 fingerbreadths above the hairline, St 1 = on the upper edge of the temporal fossa, about 4 fingerbreadths above and 1 fingerbreadth behind the angle of the orbit of the eye and cheek bone, G 14 = 2 fingerbreadths above the eyebrow on an imaginary perpendicular line through the middle of the pupil, B 2 = on the medial end of the eyebrow, G 1 = in the angle orbital curve – cheek bone, P. d. M., Point de Merveille = in the middle of the root of the nose – **(b)** – G 8 = approx. 1 fingerbreadth above the tip of the auricle and somewhat dorsal to that line, G 17 = 3 finger-breadths lateral to the midline of the skull, above the highest point of the auricle.

55

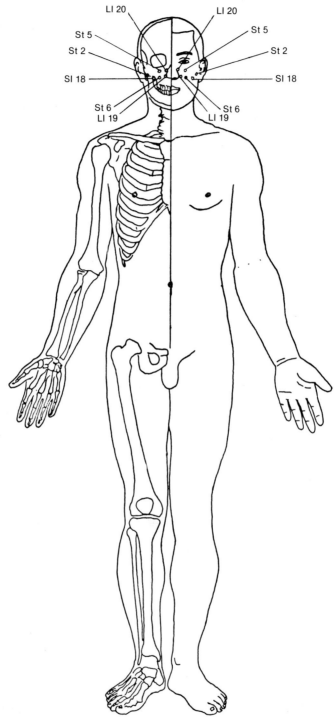

Fig. 36: Trigeminal Nerve, 2nd Branch. St 2, SI 18, LI 19, 20; St 5, 6 − St 2 = in the middle of the attachment of the masseter on the cheek bone, St 6 = on an imaginary perpendicular line through the middle of the pupil on the level of the nostril, LI 20 = on the upper end of the nasolabial groove, LI 19 = on the nasolabial groove on the level of the nostrils, SI 18 = on the anterior point of attachment of the masseter to the cheek bone in the angle these form.

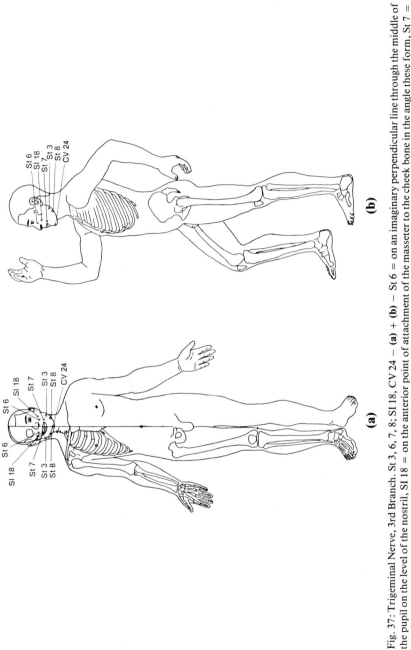

(a)

(b)

Fig. 37: Trigeminal Nerve, 3rd Branch. St 3, 6, 7, 8; SI 18, CV 24 – **(a)** + **(b)** – St 6 = on an imaginary perpendicular line through the middle of the pupil on the level of the nostril, SI 18 = on the anterior point of attachment of the masseter to the cheek bone in the angle these form, St 7 = point of intersection of an imaginary perpendicular line through the middle of the pupil and the corner of the mouth, St 3 = somewhat in front of the angle of the mandible, St 8 = on the point of intersection of an imaginary perpendicular line through the middle of the pupil and the lower edge of the mandible, CV 24 = tip of the chin.

57

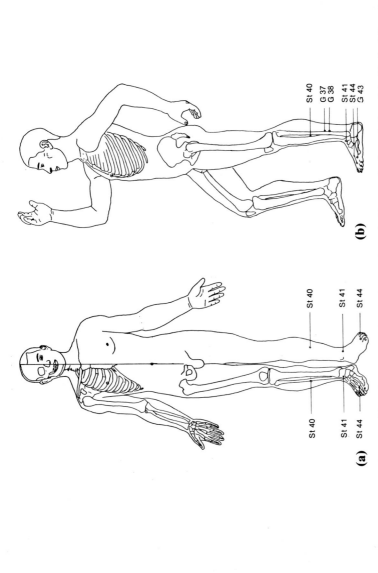

St 40
St 41
St 44

(a)

St 40
G 37
G 38

St 41
St 44
G 43

(b)

Fig. 38: Trigeminal Neuralgia, Opposition. St 40, 41, 44; G 37, 38, 43 – **(a)** – St 40 = on the frontal edge of the fibula, 1 fingerbreadth above the midpoint between the anterior tibial tubercle and the lateral malleolus, St 41 = on the lower edge of the tibia, in the middle of the tarsus, St 44 = proximal, in the angle of the metatarsophalangeal joints of the 2nd and 3rd toes – **(b)** – St 40 = on the frontal edge of the fibula, 1 fingerbreadth above the midpoint between the anterior tibial tubercle and the lateral malleolus, G 37 = 3 fingerbreadths below the midpoint between the upper edge of the tibia and the lateral malleolus, G 38 = 5 fingerbreadths above the tip of the outer ankle, on the frontal edge of the fibula, just below G 37, G 43 = on the lateral side of the metatarsophalangeal joint of the 4th toe.

58

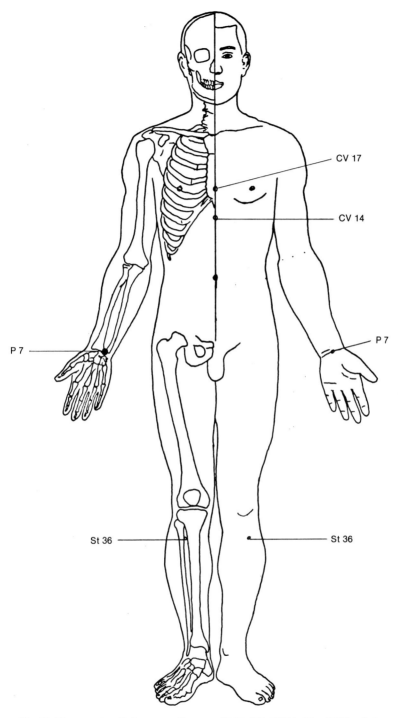

Fig. 39: Hypertension, Influence on Pressure. St 36, P 7, CV 14, 17 – St 36 = between the
m. tibialis anterior and m. extensor digit. longus, P 7 = in the middle of the largest crease
of the wrist on the volar side, CV 14 = one eighth below the xiphoid, CV 17 = on the
middle of the sternum on the level of the 4th intercostal space.

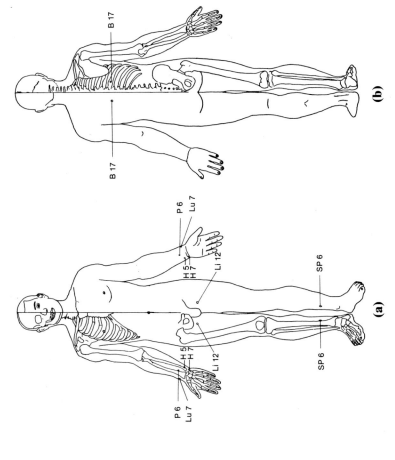

60

Fig. 40: Hypertension, Blood Flow. SP 6, P 6, Li 12, B 17, H 5, 7; Lu 7 – **(a)** – SP 6 = point of intersection, approx. 4 fingerbreadths above the lateral malleolus, P 6 = on the volar midline of the lower arm, approx. 3 fingerbreadths above the largest crease of the wrist, Li 12 = in the distal angle of Scarpa's triangle, H 5 = above the ulnar artery on the level of the ulnar apophysis, H 7 = on the radial side of the pisiform bone, Lu 7 = just 1 fingerbreadth proximal to the capitulum of the radius – **(b)** – B 17 = between the 7th and 8th thoracic vertebrae.

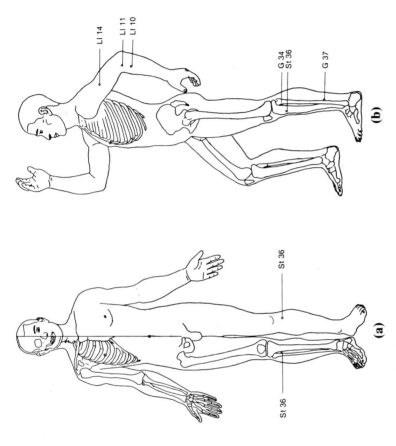

Fig. 41: Hypertension, Musculature. G 34, 37; St 36, LI 10, 11; infrequently 14 – **(a)** – St 36 = between the m. tibialis anterior and m. extensor digit. longus – **(b)** – LI 14 = on the lowest point of attachment of the deltoid muscle on the upper arm, LI 11 = on the lateral end of the crease of the elbow, LI 10 = 2 fingerbreadths distal to LI 11, G 34 = in front of and below the capitulum of the fibula, G 37 = 3 fingerbreadths below the midpoint between the upper edge of the tibia and the lateral malleolus.

62

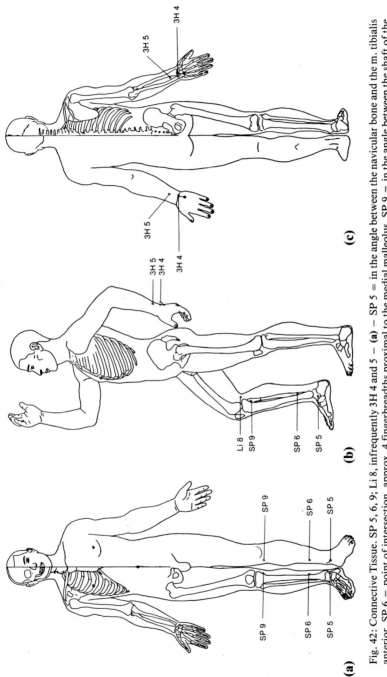

Fig. 42: Connective Tissue. SP 5, 6, 9; Li 8, infrequently 3H 4 and 5 – (a) – SP 5 = in the angle between the navicular bone and the m. tibialis anterior, SP 6 = point of intersection, approx. 4 fingerbreadths proximal to the medial malleolus, SP 9 = in the angle between the shaft of the tibia and the medial condyle – (b) – Li 8 = on the medial end of the crease of the joint of the knee, when the knee is maximally bent – (c) – 3H 5 = just 3 fingerbreadths above the capitulum of the radius, 3H 4 = on the back of the hand on the joint cavity between the hamate and the 4th metacarpal bones.

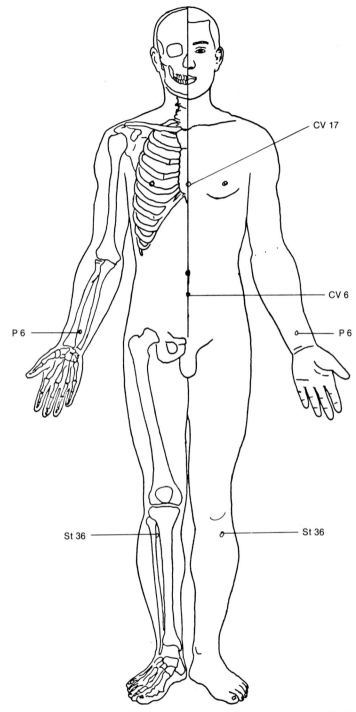

Fig. 43: Low Blood Pressure, Influence on Pressure. St 36, P 6, CV 6, 17 — St 36 = between the m. tibialis anterior and m. extensor digit. longus, P 6 = in the volar midline of the lower arm, approx. 3 fingerbreadths above the largest crease of the wrist, CV 6 = 2 fingerbreadths below the navel, CV 17 = in the middle of the sternum on the level of the 4th intercostal space.

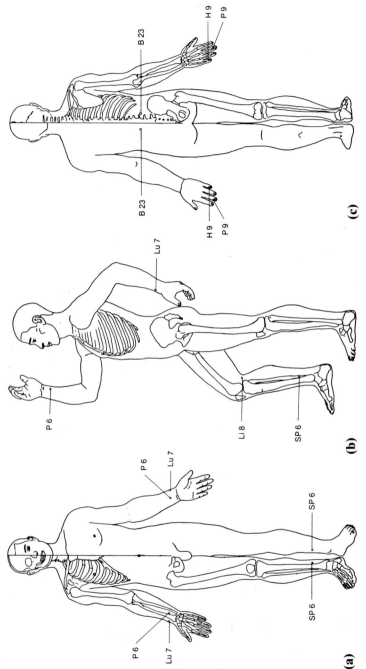

64

Fig. 44: Low Blood Pressure, Blood Flow. SP 6, P 6, Lu 7, H 9, P 9, Li 8, B 23 – **(a)** – P 6 = in the volar midline of the lower arm, approx. 3 fingerbreadths above the largest crease of the wrist, Lu 7 = just 1 fingerbreadth proximal to the capitulum of the radius, SP 6 = point of intersection, approx. 4 fingerbreadths proximal to the medial malleolus – **(b)** – Li 8 = on the medial end of the crease of the knee, when the knee is maximally bent – **(c)** – B 23 = between the 2nd and 3rd lumbar vertebrae, H 9 = approx. 2 mm medial and proximal to the corner of the cuticle of the small finger, thumb side, P 9 = approx. 2 mm medial and proximal to the corner of the cuticle of the middle finger.

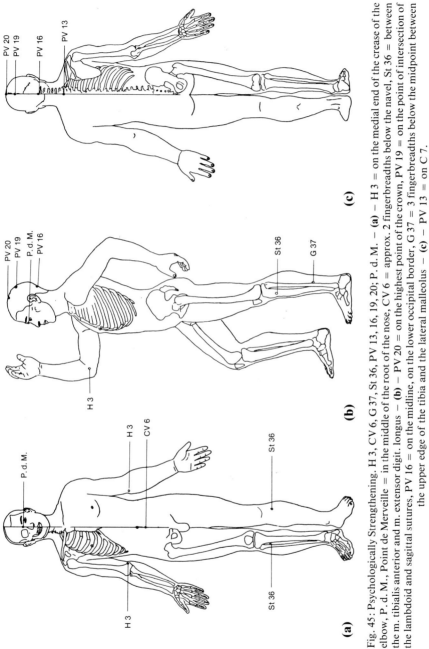

Fig. 45: Psychologically Strengthening. H 3, CV 6, G 37, St 36, PV 13, 16, 19, 20; P. d. M. – **(a)** – H 3 = on the medial end of the crease of the elbow, P. d. M., Point de Merveille = in the middle of the root of the nose, CV 6 = approx. 2 fingerbreadths below the navel, St 36 = between the m. tibialis anterior and m. extensor digit. longus – **(b)** – PV 20 = on the highest point of the crown, PV 19 = on the point of intersection of the lambdoid and sagittal sutures, PV 16 = on the midline, on the lower occipital border, G 37 = 3 fingerbreadths below the midpoint between the upper edge of the tibia and the lateral malleolus – **(c)** – PV 13 = on C 7.

65

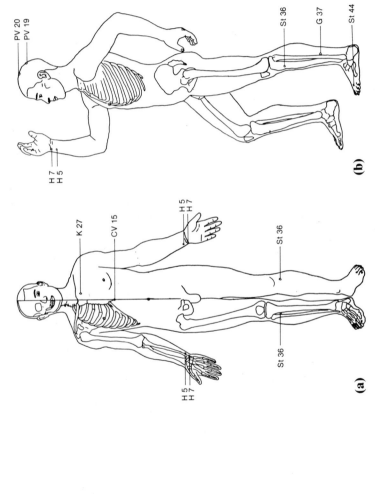

(a)

PV 20
PV 19

H 7
H 5

St 36

G 37

St 44

(b)

K 27

CV 15

H 5
H 7

St 36

H 5
H 7

St 36

Fig. 46: Psychologically Sedating. H 5, 7; St 36, 44; G 37, K 27 on the left side, CV 15, PV 19, 20 – **(a)** – K 27 = on the edge of the sternum, on the lower part of the sternoclavicular joint, CV 15 = below the tip of the xiphoid, H 5 = over the ulnar artery on the level of the ulnar apophysis, H 7 = just 1 fingerbreadth proximal to the capitulum of the radius, St 36 = between the m. tibialis anterior and m. extensor digit. longus – **(b)** – PV 20 = on the highest point of the crown, PV 19 = on the point of intersection of the lambdoid and sagittal sutures, H 7 = just 1 fingerbreadth proximal to the capitulum of the radius, H 5 = over the ulnar artery on the level of the ulnar apophysis, G 37 = 3 fingerbreadths below the midpoint between the upper edge of the tibia and the lateral malleolus, St 44 = proximal, in the angle of the metatarsophalangeal joints of the 2nd and 3rd toes.

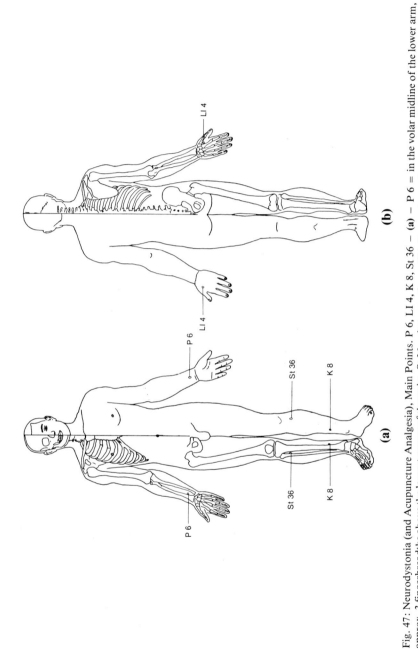

(b)

(a)

Fig. 47: Neurodystonia (and Acupuncture Analgesia), Main Points. P 6, LI 4, K 8, St 36 – **(a)** – P 6 = in the volar midline of the lower arm, approx. 3 fingerbreadths above the largest crease of the wrist, St 36 = between the m. tibialis anterior and m. extensor digit. longus, K 8 = point of intersection with SP 6 and Li 5; approx. 4 fingerbreadths proximal to the internal malleolus – **(b)** – LI 4 = in the proximal angle between the 1st and 2nd metacarpal bones.

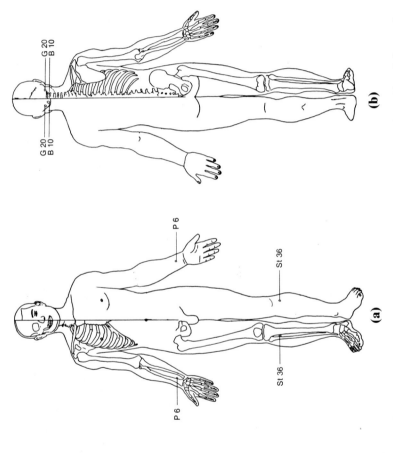

Fig. 48: Neurodystonia (and Acupuncture Analgesia), Basic Regulation. B 10, G 20, P 6, St 36 – **(a)** – P 6 = on the volar midline of the lower arm, approx. 3 fingerbreadths above the largest crease of the wrist, St 36 = between the m. tibialis anterior and m. extensor digit. longus – **(b)** – G 20 = on the lower occipital border, just behind the mastoid, B 10 = on the lower edge of the squama occipitalis, 2 fingerbreadths lateral to the dorsal midline.

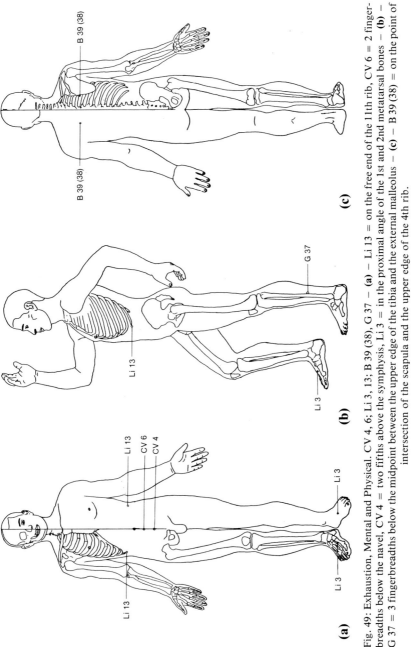

Fig. 49: Exhaustion, Mental and Physical. CV 4, 6; Li 3, 13; B 39 (38), G 37 – **(a)** – Li 13 = on the free end of the 11th rib, CV 6 = 2 fingerbreadths below the navel, CV 4 = two fifths above the symphysis, Li 3 = in the proximal angle of the 1st and 2nd metatarsal bones – **(b)** – G 37 = 3 fingerbreadths below the midpoint between the upper edge of the tibia and the external malleolus – **(c)** – B 39 (38) = on the point of intersection of the scapula and the upper edge of the 4th rib.

69

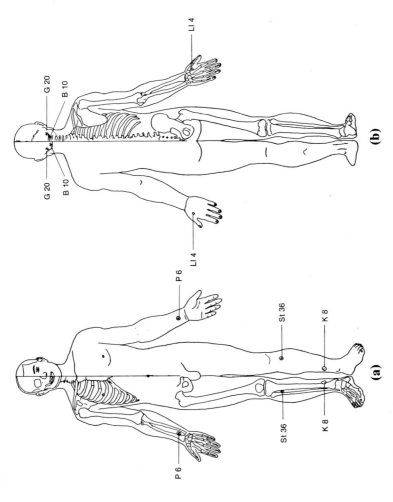

(a)

(b)

Fig. 50: Neurasthenia, Basic Regulation (B 10, G 20, St 36, P 6) and/or Main Points (P 6, LI 4, K 8, St 36) – **(a)** – P 6 = on the volar midline of the lower arm, approx. 3 fingerbreadths above the largest crease of the wrist, St 36 = between the m. tibialis anterior and m. extensor digit. longus, K 8 = point of intersection, approx. 4 fingerbreadths proximal to the internal malleolus – **(b)** – G 20 = on the lower occipital border, just behind the mastoid, B 10 = on the lower edge of the squama occipitalis, 2 fingerbreadths lateral to the dorsal midline, LI 4 = in the proximal angle between the 1st and 2nd metacarpal bones.

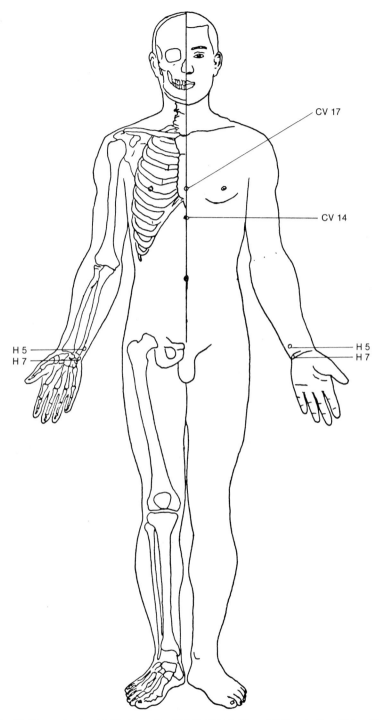

Fig. 51: Neurasthenia with Tachycardia. H 5, 7; CV 14, 17 − CV 17 = in the middle of the sternum on the level of the 4th intercostal space, H 5 = over the ulnar artery on the level of the ulnar apophysis, H 7 = on the radial side of the pisiform bone, CV 14 = one eighth below the xiphoid.

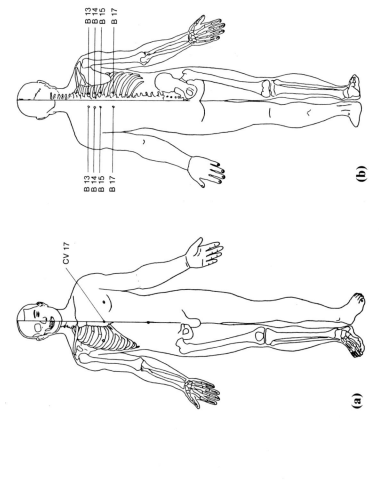

(a)

CV 17

(b)

B 13
B 14
B 15
B 17

B 13
B 14
B 15
B 17

Fig. 52: Neurasthenia with Disorders in the Thorax. B 13, 14, 15, 17; CV 17 − **(a)** − B 13 = between the 3rd and 4th thoracic vertebrae (Lu*), B 14 = between the 4th and 5th thoracic vertebrae (P), B 15 = between the 5th and 6th thoracic vertebrae (H), B 17 = between the 7th and 8th thoracic vertebrae (diaphragm) − **(b)** − CV 17 = in the middle of the sternum on the level of the 4th intercostal space.
*The organ, Lung, in parenthesis means that point of the Bladder Meridian is the associated (concurring) point of the Lung. See also "The Specific Types of Acupuncture Points".

72

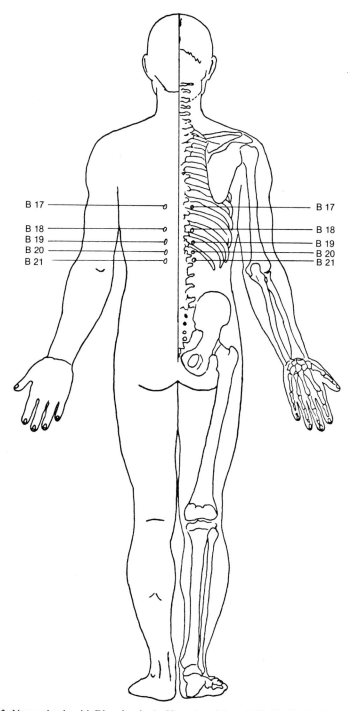

B 17 ——————o   o—————— B 17
B 18 —————o   o————— B 18
B 19 —————o   o————— B 19
B 20 ————o   o———— B 20
B 21 ————o   o———— B 21

Fig. 53: Neurasthenia with Disorders in the Hypochondrium. B 17, 18, 19, 20, 21 – B 17 = between the 7th and 8th thoracic vertebrae (diaphragm), B 18 = between the 9th and 10th thoracic vertebrae (Li), B 19 = between the 10th and 11th thoracic vertebrae (G), B 20 = between the 11th and 12th thoracic vertebrae (SP), B 21 = between the 12th thoracic and 1st lumbar vertebrae (St).

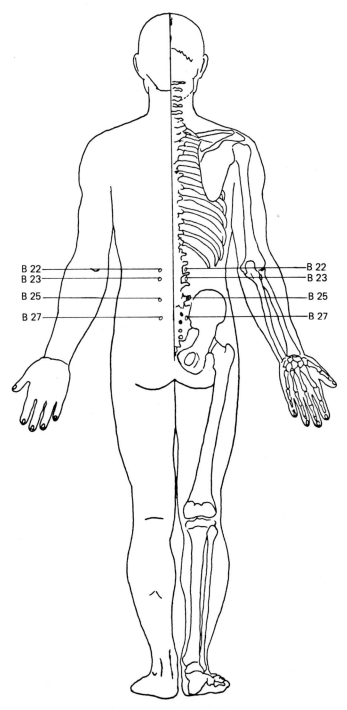

Fig. 54: Neurasthenia with Disorders of the Excretory Organs. B 22, 23, 25, 27 – B 22 = between the 1st and 2nd lumbar vertebrae (3H), B 23 = between the 2nd and 3rd lumbar vertebrae (K), B 25 = between the 4th and 5th lumbar vertebrae (LI), B 27 = on the posterior superior iliac spine (SI).

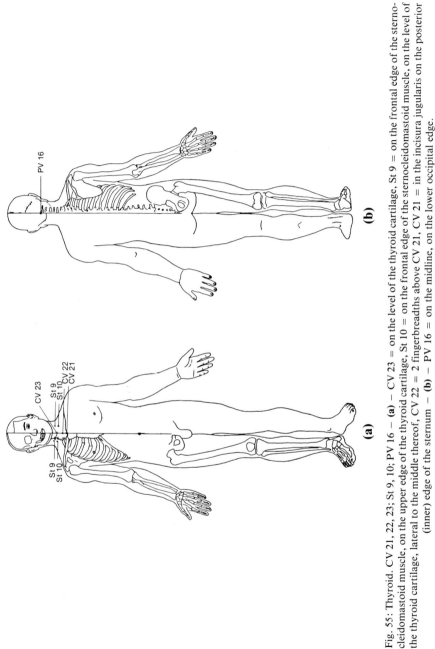

Fig. 55: Thyroid. CV 21, 22, 23; St 9, 10; PV 16 – **(a)** – CV 23 = on the level of the thyroid cartilage, St 9 = on the frontal edge of the sterno-cleidomastoid muscle, on the upper edge of the thyroid cartilage, St 10 = on the frontal edge of the sternocleidomastoid muscle, on the level of the thyroid cartilage, lateral to the middle thereof, CV 22 = 2 fingerbreadths above CV 21, CV 21 = in the incisura jugularis on the posterior (inner) edge of the sternum – **(b)** – PV 16 = on the midline, on the lower occipital edge.

75

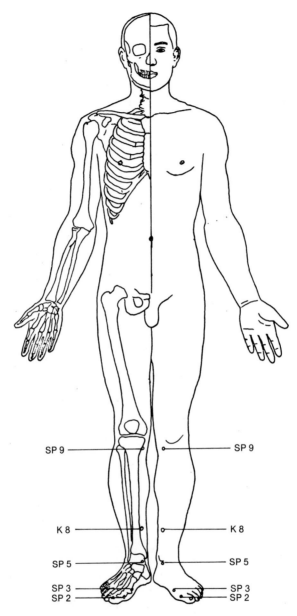

Fig. 56: Pickwickian Syndrome. SP 2, 3, 5, 9; K 8 – SP 9 = in the angle between the shaft of the tibia and the medial condyle, K 8 = point of intersection, approx. 4 fingerbreadths proximal to the medial malleolus, SP 5 = in the angle between the navicular bone and the m. tibialis anterior, SP 3 = on the tendon of the hallucal abductor on the inner edge of the foot, just proximal to the metatarsophalangeal joint of the big toe, SP 2 = on the medial side of the articulation of the metatarsophalangeal joint of the big toe.

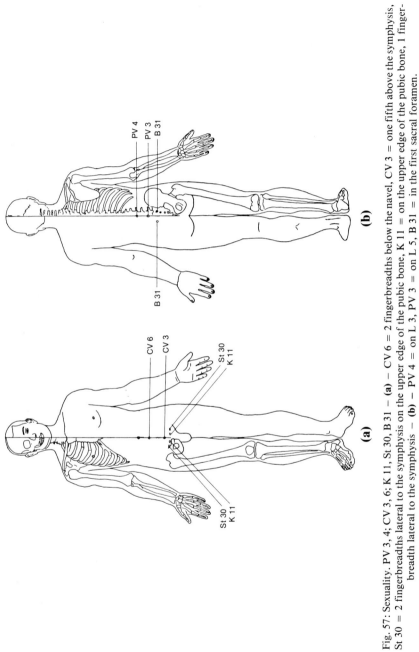

Fig. 57: Sexuality. PV 3, 4; CV 3, 6; K 11, St 30, B 31 – (a) – CV 6 = 2 fingerbreadths below the navel, CV 3 = one fifth above the symphysis, St 30 = 2 fingerbreadths lateral to the symphysis on the upper edge of the pubic bone, K 11 = on the upper edge of the pubic bone, 1 fingerbreadth lateral to the symphysis – (b) – PV 4 = on L 3, PV 3 = on L 5, B 31 = in the first sacral foramen.

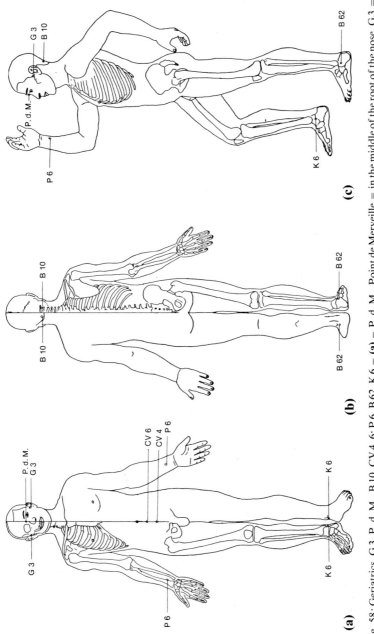

(a)

(b)

(c)

Fig. 58: Geriatrics. G 3, P. d. M., B 10, CV 4, 6; P 6, B 62, K 6 – **(a)** – P. d. M., Point de Merveille = in the middle of the root of the nose, G 3 = just above the middle of the cheek bone, CV 6 = 2 fingerbreadths below the navel, CV 4 = two fifths above the symphysis – **(b)** – B 10 = on the lower edge of the squama occipitalis, 2 fingerbreadths lateral to the dorsal midline, B 62 = 2 fingerbreadths below the distal tip of the external malleolus – **(c)** – P 6 = on the volar midline of the lower arm, approx. 3 fingerbreadths above the largest crease of the wrist, K 6 = 1 fingerbreadth beneath the internal malleolus.

78

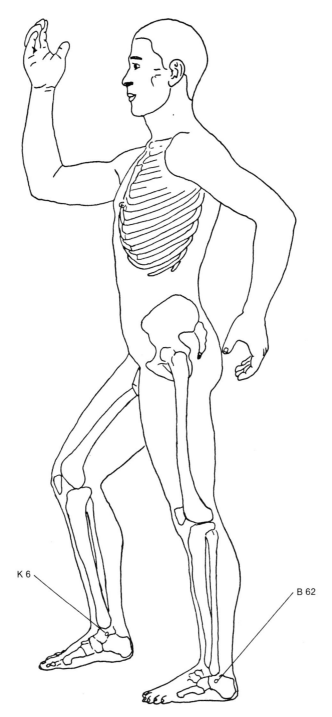

Fig. 59: Sleep, in general. B 62, K 6 — B 62 = 2 fingerbreadths below the distal tip of the external malleolus, K 6 = 1 fingerbreadth below the internal malleolus.

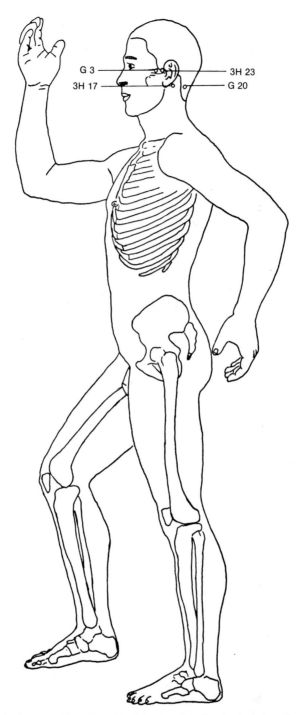

Fig. 60: Vertigo, otogenic. 3H 17, 23; G 3, 20 − 3H 23 = in the indentation between the tragus and the upper point of attachment of the auricle, G 3 = just above the middle of the cheek bone, 3H 17 = on the frontal edge of the mastoid, behind the lobe of the ear, G 20 = on the lower occipital border, just behind the mastoid.

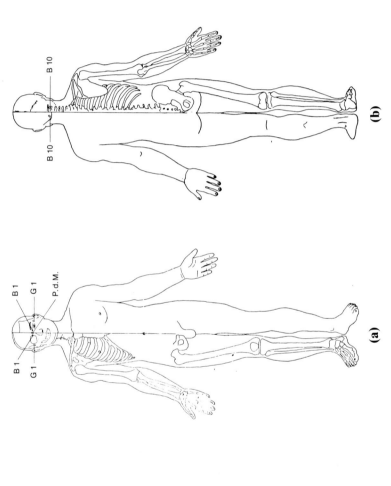

(a)

(b)

Fig. 61: Vertigo, ophthalmic. B 1, 10; P. d. M., G 1 – **(a)** – B 1 = in the medial angle of the orbit, G 1 = in the angle orbital curve – cheek bone, P. d. M., Point de Merveille = in the middle of the root of the nose – **(b)** – B 10 = on the lower edge of the squama occipitalis, 2 finger-breadths lateral to the dorsal midline.

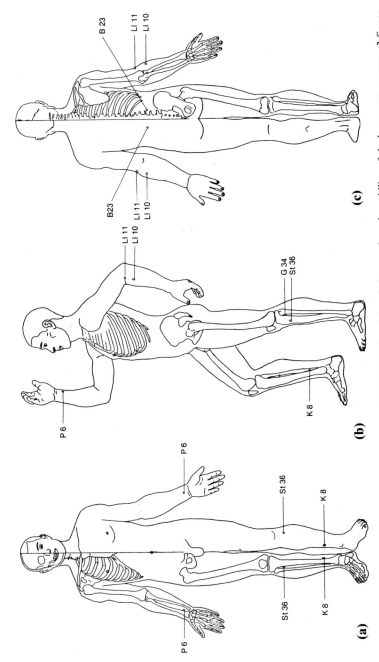

82

Fig. 62: Musculature, general. G 34, St 36, LI 10, 11; K 8, P 6, B 23 – (a) – P 6 = on the volar midline of the lower arm, approx. 3 finger-breadths above the largest crease of the wrist, St 36 = between the m. tibialis anterior and m. extensor digit. longus, K 8 = point of intersection, approx. 4 fingerbreadths proximal to the medial malleolus – (b) – LI 11 = on the lateral end of the crease of the elbow, LI 10 = 2 finger-breadths distal to LI 11, G 34 = in front of and distal to the capitulum of the fibula, K 8 = point of intersection, approx. 4 fingerbreadths proxi-mal to the medial malleolus – (c) – B 23 = between the 2nd and 3rd lumbar vertebrae (associated point of the Kidney).

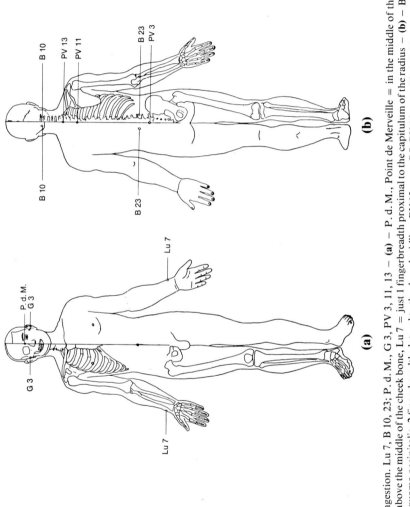

(b)

(a)

Fig. 63: Congestion. Lu 7, B 10, 23; P. d. M., G 3, PV 3, 11, 13 – **(a)** – P. d. M., Point de Merveille = in the middle of the root of the nose, G 3 = just above the middle of the cheek bone, Lu 7 = just 1 fingerbreadth proximal to the capitulum of the radius – **(b)** – B 10 = on the lower edge of the squama occipitalis, 2 fingerbreadths lateral to the dorsal midline, PV 13 = on C 7, PV 11 = on Th 4, B 23 = between the 2nd and 3rd lumbar vertebrae (associated point of the Kidney), PV 3 = on the tip of the spinous process of L 5.

83

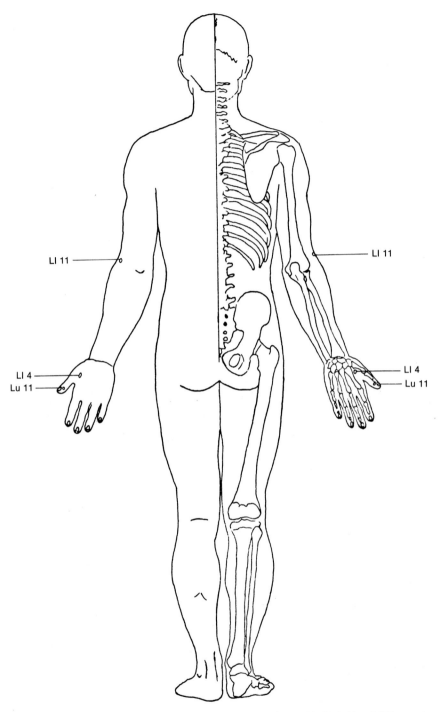

Fig. 64: Disorders of the Throat, general (basic framework). Lu 11, LI 4, 11 − LI 11 = on the lateral end of the crease of the elbow, LI 4 = in the proximal angle between the 1st and 2nd metacarpal bones, Lu 11 = 2 mm proximal and lateral to the cuticle of the thumb on the index finger side.

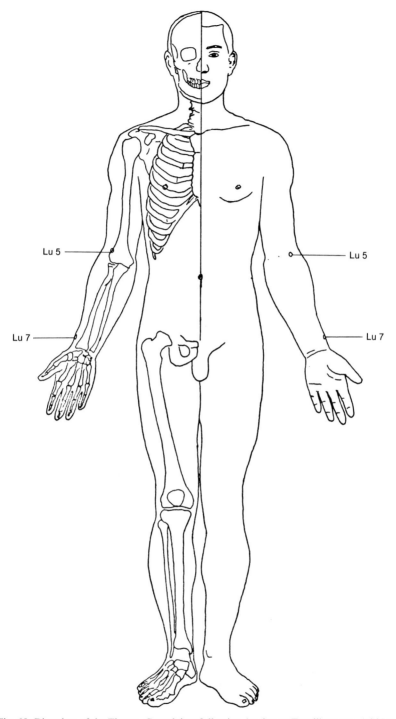

Lu 5

Lu 5

Lu 7

Lu 7

Fig. 65: Disorders of the Throat, Complaints following Angina or Tonsillectomy. Add Lu 5, 7 − Lu 5 = on the lateral border of the biceps tendon, in the middle of the crease of the elbow, Lu 7 = just 1 fingerbreadth proximal to the capitulum of the radius.

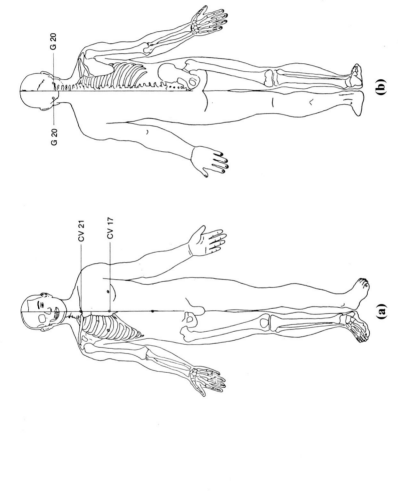

Fig. 66: Disorders of the Throat, Pharyngitis. Add CV 17, 21; G 20 – **(a)** – CV 21 = in the incisura jugularis on the posterior (inner) edge of the sternum, CV 17 = in the middle of the sternum on the level of the 4th intercostal space – **(b)** – G 20 = on the lower occipital border, just behind the mastoid.

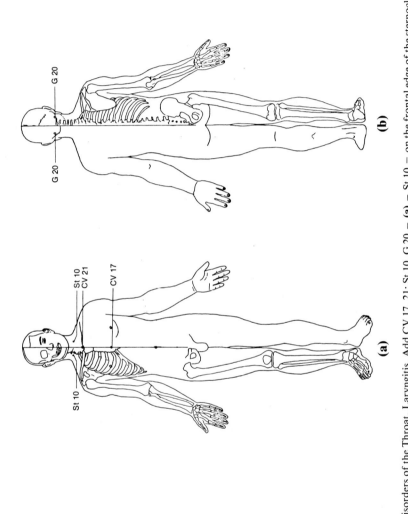

Fig. 67: Disorders of the Throat, Laryngitis. Add CV 17, 21; St 10, G 20 – (a) – St 10 = on the frontal edge of the sternocleidomastoid m. on the level of the thyroid cartilage, lateral to the center thereof, CV 21 = in the incisura jugularis on the posterior (inner) sider of the sternum, CV 17 = in the middle of the sternum on the level of the 4th intercostal space – (b) – G 20 = on the lower occipital border, just behind the mastoid.

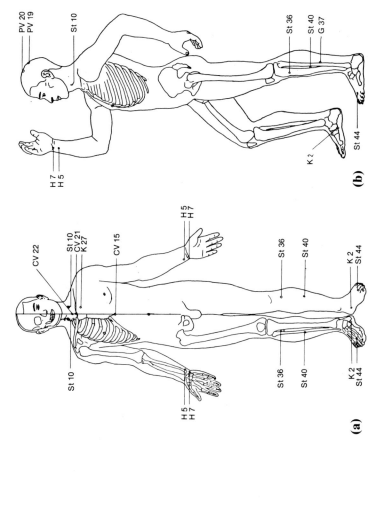

(a)

PV 20
PV 19

St 10

St 36

St 40

G 37

K 2

St 44

(b)

H 7
H 5

CV 22

St 10
CV 21
K 27

CV 15

St 10

H 5
H 7

St 36

St 40

K 2
St 44

H 5
H 7

St 36

St 40

K 2
St 44

Fig. 68: Disorders of the Throat, Spastic Aphonia. Add CV 15, 21, 22; H 5/7, St 10, 36, 40, 44; K 2, 27 on the left side, PV 19/20, G 37 – **(a)** – CV 22 = 2 fingerbreadths above CV 21, St 10 = on the frontal edge of the sternocleidomastoid m. on the level of the thyroid cartilage, lateral to the center thereof, CV 21 = in the incisura jugularis on the posterior (inner) side of the sternum, K 27 = on the edge of the sternum, on the lower part of the sternoclavicular joint, CV 15 = below the tip of the xiphoid, H 5 = on the level of the ulnar apophysis, H 7 = on the radial side of the pisiform bone, St 36 = between the m. tibialis anterior and m. extensor digit. longus, St 40 = on the frontal edge of the fibula, 1 fingerbreadth above the midpoint between the anterior tibial tubercle and the lateral malleolus, K 2 = just below the protrusion of the navicular bone, St 44 = proximal, in the angle of the metatarsophalangeal joints of the 1st and 2nd toes – **(b)** – PV 20 = on the highest point of the crown, PV 19 = on the point of intersection of the lambdoid and sagittal sutures, G 37 = 3 fingerbreadths below the midpoint between the upper edge of the tibia and the lateral malleolus.

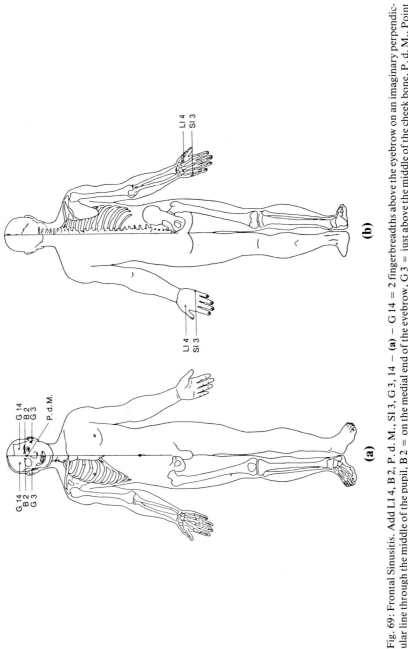

(a)

G 14
B 2
G 3
P. d. M.

G 14
B 2
G 3

(b)

LI 4
SI 3

LI 4
SI 3

Fig. 69: Frontal Sinusitis. Add LI 4, B 2, P. d. M., SI 3, G 3, 14 – **(a)** – G 14 = 2 fingerbreadths above the eyebrow on an imaginary perpendicular line through the middle of the pupil, B 2 = on the medial end of the eyebrow, G 3 = just above the middle of the cheek bone, P. d. M., Point de Merveille = in the middle of the root of the nose – **(b)** – LI 4 = in the proximal angle between the 1st and 2nd metacarpal bones, SI 3 = on the lateral end of the skin fold behind (proximal to) the metacarpophalangeal joint of the small finger, when the hand is closed in a fist.

89

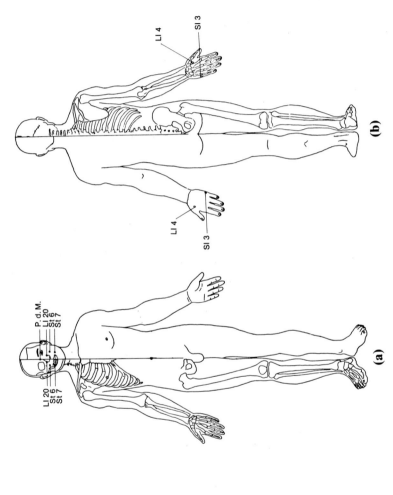

(b)

(a)

Fig. 70: Maxillary Sinusitis. Add LI 4, 20; SI 3, St 6, 7; P. d. M. – **(a)** – P. d. M., Point de Merveille = in the middle of the root of the nose, LI 20 = on the upper end of the nasolabial groove, St 6 = on an imaginary perpendicular line through the middle of the pupil on the level of the nostril, St 7 = point of intersection of an imaginary perpendicular line through the middle of the pupil and the corner of the mouth – **(b)** – LI 4 = in the proximal angle between the 1st and 2nd metacarpal bones, SI 3 = on the lateral end of the skin fold behind (proximal to) the metacarpophalangeal joint of the small finger, when the hand is closed in a fist.

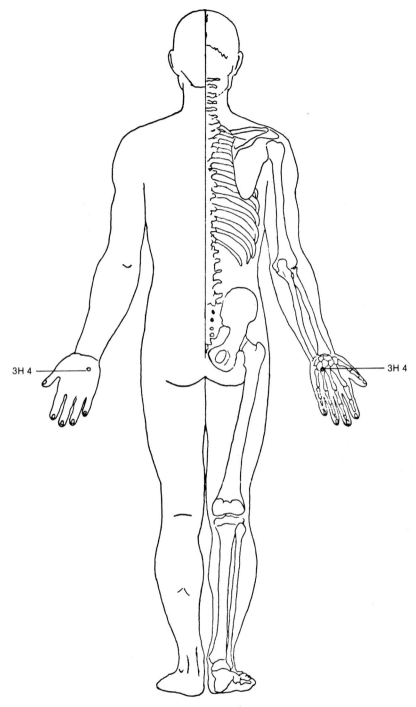

3H 4

3H 4

Fig. 71: Vasomotor Rhinitis. Add 3 H 4 − 3 H 4 = between the hamate and 4th metacarpal bones.

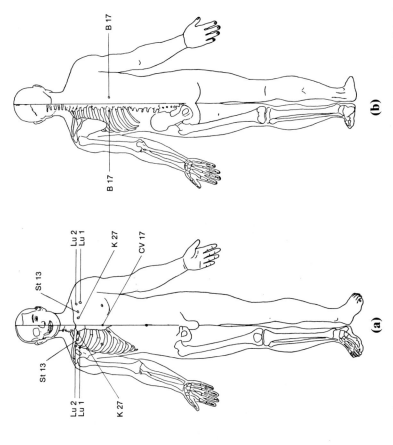

(a)

St 13

Lu 2
Lu 1

K 27

CV 17

St 13

Lu 2
Lu 1

K 27

B 17

B 17

(b)

Fig. 72: Bronchial Spasms. CV 17, Lu 1, 2; K 27, St 13, B 17 – **(a)** – St 13 = like St 12, but on the lower edge of the clavicula, Lu 2 = like Lu 1, but in the 2nd intercostal space, Lu 1 = on the frontal axillary line on the level of the 3rd intercostal space, K 27 = on the edge of the sternum, on the lateral part of the sternoclavicular joint, CV 17 = in the middle of the sternum on the level of the 4th intercostal space – **(b)** – B 17 = on the level of Th 7 (associated point of the diaphragm).

92

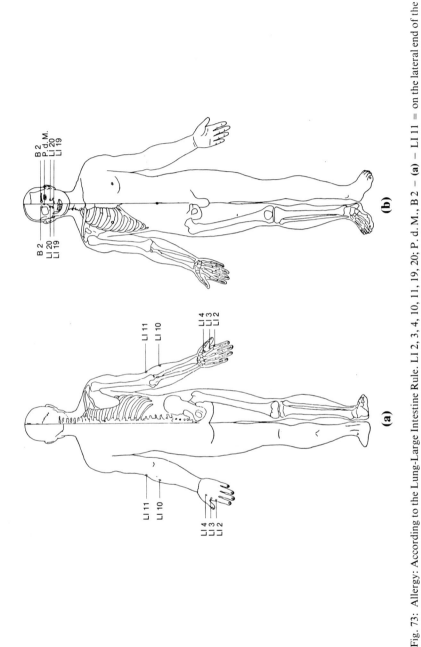

Fig. 73: Allergy: According to the Lung-Large Intestine Rule. LI 2, 3, 4, 10, 11, 19, 20; P. d. M., B 2 – **(a)** – LI 11 = on the lateral end of the crease of the elbow, LI 10 = 2 fingerbreadths distal to LI 11, LI 4 = in the proximal angle between the 1st and 2nd metacarpal bones, LI 3 = immediately proximal to the joint cavity of the metacarpophalangeal joint of the index finger, LI 2 = just distal to the metacarpophalangeal joint of the index finger – **(b)** – B 2 = on the medial end of the eyebrow, P. d. M., Point de Merveille = in the middle of the root of the nose, LI 20 = on the upper end of the nasolabial groove, LI 19 = in the nasolabial groove on the level of the nostril.

93

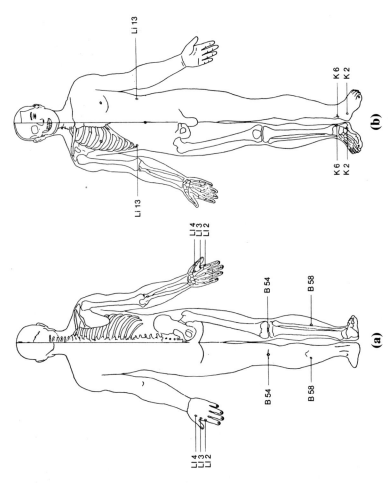

(b)

(a)

94

Fig. 74: Allergy: With Metabolic Points. B 54, 58; K 2, 6; Li 13, LI 2, 3, 4 – **(a)** – LI 4 = in the proximal angle between the 1st and 2nd metacarpal bones, LI 3 = immediately proximal to the joint cavity of the metacarpophalangeal joint of the index finger, LI 2 = just distal to the metacarpophalangeal joint of the index finger, B 54 = in the middle of the popliteal space, B 58 = on the outer side of the calf – **(b)** – Li 13 = on the free end of the 11th rib, K 6 = 1 fingerbreadth below the internal malleolus, K 2 = just below the protrusion of the navicular bone.

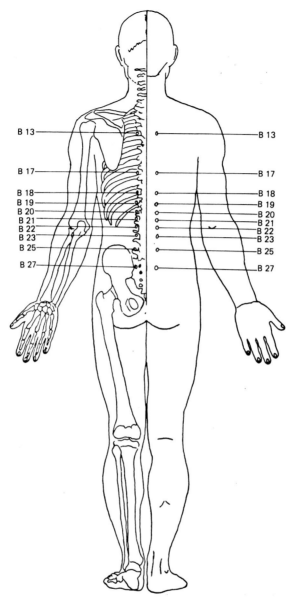

Fig. 75: Allergy: With Associated (Concurring) Points. B 13, 17, 18, 19, 20, 21, 22, 23, 25, 27 – B 13 = on the level of Th 3 (associated point of the Lung), B 17 = on the level of Th 7 (associated point of the diaphragm), B 18 = on the level of Th 9 (associated point of the Liver), B 19 = on the level of Th 10 (associated point of the Gallbladder), B 20 = on the level of Th 11 (associated point of the Spleen-Pancreas), B 21 = on the level of Th 12 (associated point of the Stomach), B 22 = on the level of L 2 (associated point of the 3H), B 23 = on the level of L 3 (associated point of the Kidney), B 25 = on the level of L 5 (associated point of the Large Intestine), B 27 = on the posterior superior iliac spine (associated point of the Small Intestine).

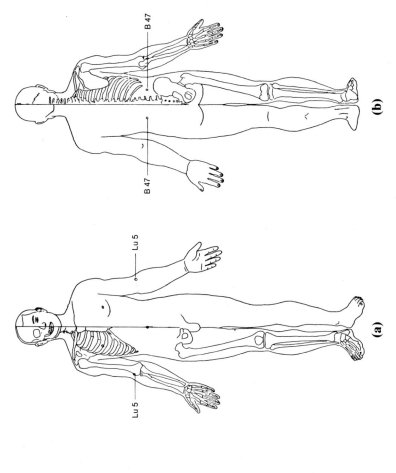

(a)

(b)

Fig. 76: Allergy: Adjuvant Points. B 47, Lu 5 – **(a)** – Lu 5 = on the lateral border of the biceps tendon, in the middle of the crease of the elbow – **(b)** – B 47 = 1 fingerbreadth above the iliac crest and 4 fingerbreadths lateral to the dorsal midline on the point of intersection of the two.

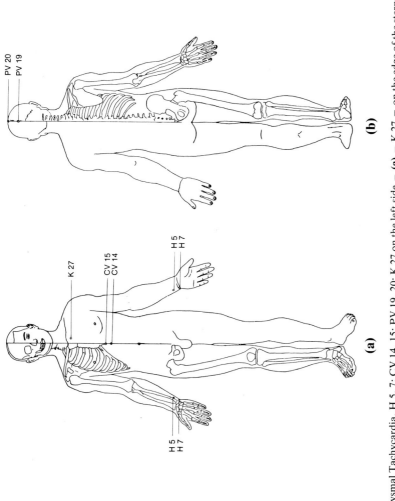

(a)

(b)

Fig. 77: Paroxysmal Tachycardia. H 5, 7; CV 14, 15; PV 19, 20; K 27 on the left side – **(a)** – K 27 = on the edge of the sternum, on the lower part of the sternoclavicular joint, CV 15 = below the tip of the xiphoid, CV 14 = one eighth below the xiphoid, H 5 = on the level of the ulnar apophysis, H 7 = on the radial side of the pisiform bone – **(b)** – PV 20 = on the highest point of the crown, PV 19 = on the point of intersection of the lambdoid and sagittal sutures.

97

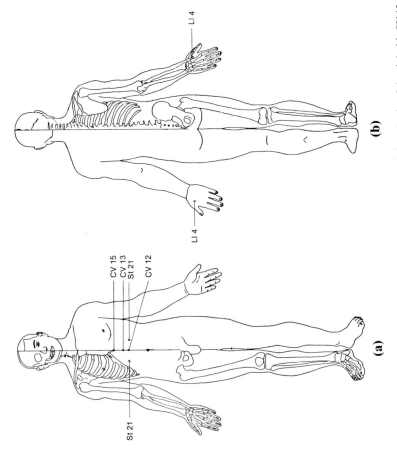

Fig. 78: Hypogastrium (see also Fig. 53). CV 12, 13, 15; LI 4, St 21 – **(a)** – CV 15 = below the tip of the xiphoid, CV 13 = three eighths below the xiphoid, CV 12 = exactly midway between the navel and the xiphoid, St 21 = in the angle of the 8th intercostal space, often 1 fingerbreadth medial thereto – **(b)** – LI 4 = in the proximal angle between the 1st and 2nd metacarpal bones.

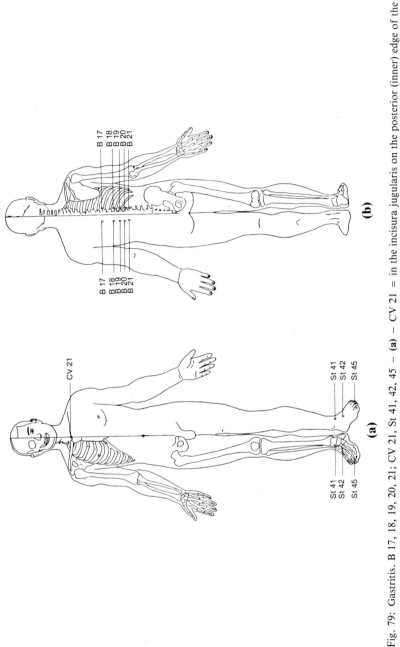

B 17
B 18
B 19
B 20
B 21

B 17
B 18
B 19
B 20
B 21

(b)

CV 21

St 41
St 42
St 45

St 41
St 42
St 45

(a)

Fig. 79: Gastritis. B 17, 18, 19, 20, 21; CV 21, St 41, 42, 45 – **(a)** – CV 21 = in the incisura jugularis on the posterior (inner) edge of the sternum, St 41 = in the middle of the tarsus, on the lower edge of the tibia, St 42 = over the joint of the navicular bone with the 2nd and 3rd cuneiform bones, St 45 = 2 mm proximal and lateral to the corner of the cuticle of the 2nd toe – **(b)** – B 17 = on the level of Th 7 (associated point of the diaphragm), B 18 = on the level of Th 9 (associated point of the Liver), B 19 = on the level of Th 10 (associated point of the Gall-bladder), B 20 = on the level of Th 11 (associated point of the Spleen-Pancreas), B 21 = on the level of Th 12 (associated point of the Stomach).

99

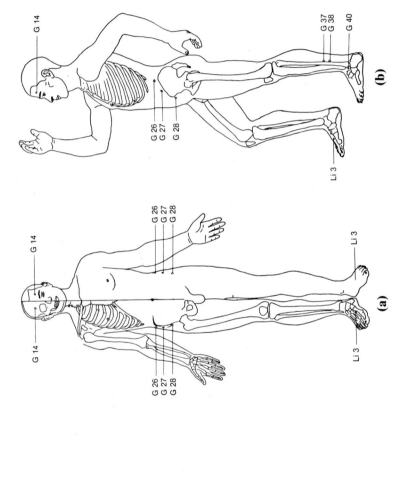

(a)

(b)

Fig. 80: Bile Flow. G 14, 26, 27, 28, 37, 38, 40; Li 3 – (a) – G 14 = 2 fingerbreadths above the eyebrow on an imaginary perpendicular line through the middle of the pupil, G 26 = on the highest point of the iliac crest, G 27 = on the iliac crest between G 26 and 28, G 28 = on the anterior superior iliac spine, Li 3 = in the proximal angle of the 1st and 2nd metatarsal bones – (b) – G 37 = 3 fingerbreadths below the midpoint between the upper edge of the tibia and the external malleolus, G 38 = 5 fingerbreadths above the tip of the external malleolus on the frontal edge of the fibula, G 40 = over the calcaneo-cuboid joint, Li 3 = in the proximal angle of the 1st and 2nd metatarsal bones.

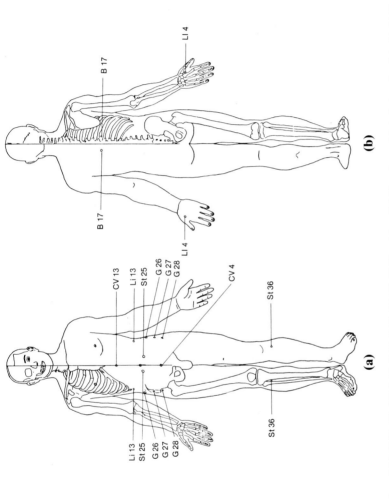

(b)

(a)

Fig. 81: Meteorism: LI 4, St 25, 36; CV 4, 13; B 17, G 26, 27, 28; Li 13 – **(a)** – CV 13 = three eighths below the xiphoid, Li 13 = on the free end of the 11th rib, St 25 = approx. 2 fingerbreadths lateral to the navel, or midway between the navel and the anterior superior iliac crest, G 26 = on the highest point of the iliac crest, G 27 = on the iliac crest between G 26 and 28, G 28 = on the anterior superior iliac spine, CV 4 = two fifths above the symphysis, St 36 = between the m. tibialis anterior and m. extensor digit. longus – **(b)** – B 17 = on the level of Th 7 (associated point of the diaphragm), LI 4 = in the proximal angle between the 1st and 2nd metacarpal bones.

101

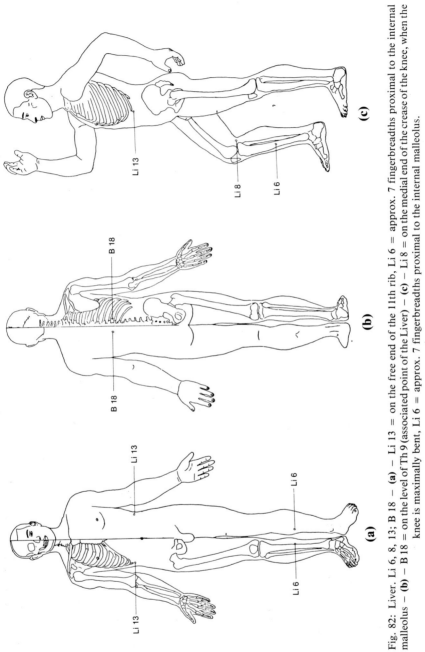

Fig. 82: Liver. Li 6, 8, 13; B 18 – **(a)** – Li 13 = on the free end of the 11th rib, Li 6 = approx. 7 fingerbreadths proximal to the internal malleolus – **(b)** – B 18 = on the level of Th 9 (associated point of the Liver) – **(c)** – Li 8 = on the medial end of the crease of the knee, when the knee is maximally bent, Li 6 = approx. 7 fingerbreadths proximal to the internal malleolus.

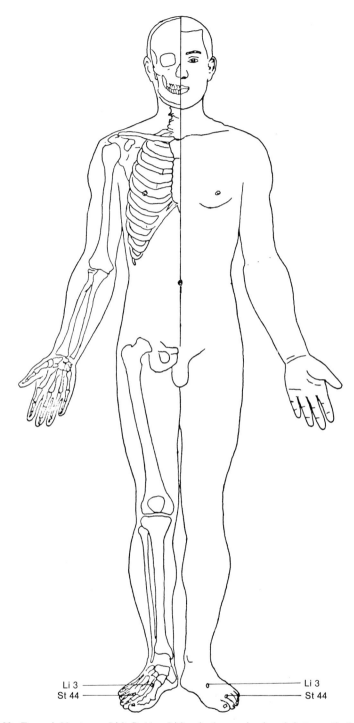

Li 3 ⎯⎯⎯⎯⎯⎯⎯⎯   ⎯⎯⎯⎯ Li 3
St 44 ⎯⎯⎯⎯⎯⎯   ⎯⎯⎯⎯ St 44

Fig. 83: Enuresis Nocturna. Li 3, St 44 − Li 3 = in the proximal angle between the 1st and 2nd metatarsal bones, St 44 = proximal, in the angle of the metatarsophalangeal joints of the 2nd and 3rd toes.

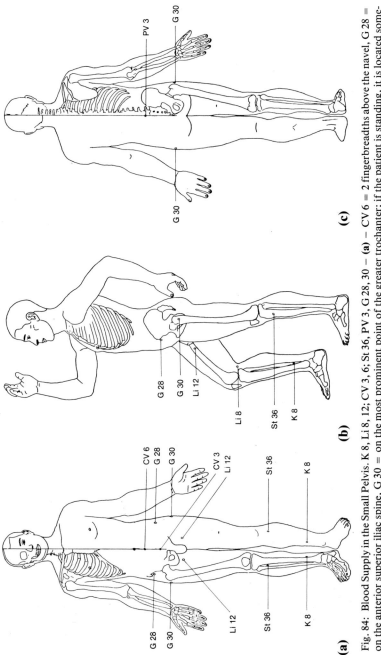

(a)

G 28
G 30

CV 6
CV 28
G 30

Li 12

CV 3
Li 12

St 36

St 36

K 8

K 8

(b)

G 28
G 30
Li 12

Li 8

St 36

K 8

(c)

PV 3
G 30

G 30

Fig. 84: Blood Supply in the Small Pelvis. K 8, Li 8, 12; CV 3, 6; St 36, PV 3, G 28, 30 – **(a)** – CV 6 = 2 fingerbreadths above the navel, G 28 = on the anterior superior iliac spine, G 30 = on the most prominent point of the greater trochanter; if the patient is standing, it is located somewhat farther dorsally, CV 3 = 2 fingerbreadths above the symphysis, Li 12 = in the distal angle of Scarpa's triangle, St 36 = between the m. tibialis anterior and m. extensor digit. longus, K 8 = point of intersection, approx. 4 fingerbreadths above the internal malleolus – **(b)** – Li 8 = on the medial end of the crease of the knee when the knee is maximally bent – **(c)** – PV 3 = on the tip of the spinous process of L 5.

104

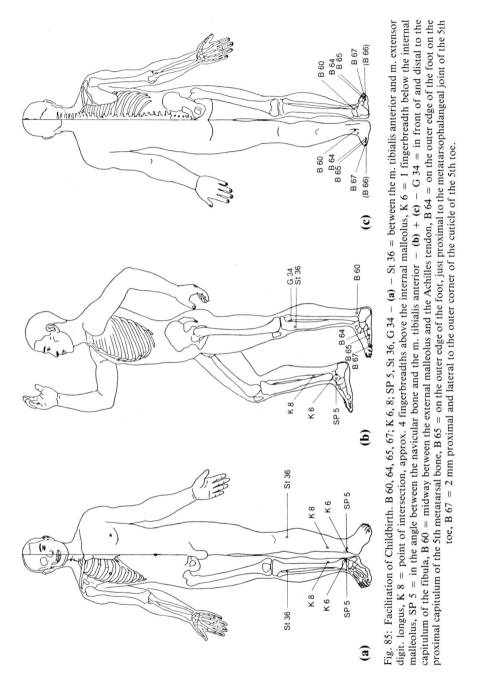

Fig. 85: Facilitation of Childbirth. B 60, 64, 65, 67; K 6, 8; SP 5, St 36, G 34 – **(a)** – St 36 = between the m. tibialis anterior and m. extensor digit. longus, K 8 = point of intersection, approx. 4 fingerbreadths above the internal malleolus, K 6 = 1 fingerbreadth below the internal malleolus, SP 5 = in the angle between the navicular bone and the m. tibialis anterior – **(b)** – G 34 = in front of and distal to the capitulum of the fibula, B 60 = midway between the external malleolus and the Achilles tendon, B 64 = on the outer edge of the foot on the proximal capitulum of the 5th metatarsal bone, B 65 = on the outer edge of the foot, just proximal to the metatarsophalangeal joint of the 5th toe, B 67 = 2 mm proximal and lateral to the outer corner of the cuticle of the 5th toe.

105

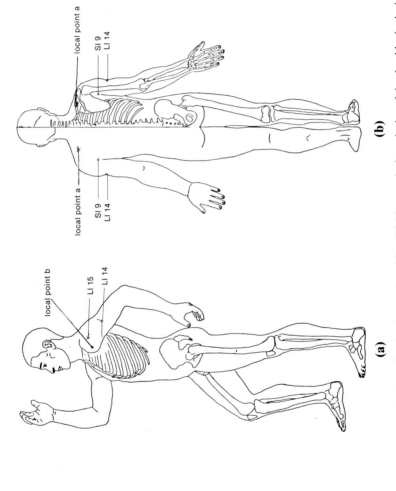

(a)

(b)

Fig. 86: Shoulder. LI 14, 15; SI 9, two local points, a, b – **(a)** – LI 15 = on the lateral edge of the shoulder in the indentation beneath the acromion, LI 14 = on the lowest point of attachment of the deltoid m. on the upper arm – **(b)** – SI 9 = 2 fingerbreadths above the dorsal end of the axillary fold, two local points: a) plainly palpable point on the m. supraspinatus, b) across from SI 9, however, higher, in a 30° ventral angle.

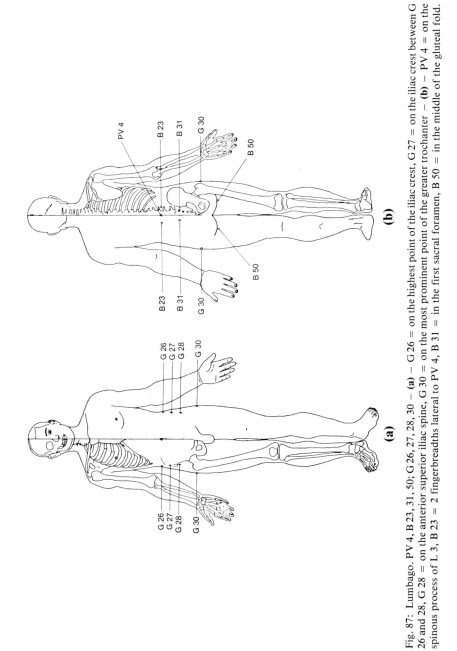

Fig. 87: Lumbago. PV 4, B 23, 31, 50; G 26, 27, 28, 30 – **(a)** – G 26 = on the highest point of the iliac crest between G 26 and 28, G 27 = on the iliac crest between G 26 and 28, G 27 = on the most prominent point of the greater trochanter – **(b)** – PV 4 = on the spinous process of L 3, B 23 = 2 fingerbreadths lateral to PV 4, B 31 = in the first sacral foramen, B 50 = in the middle of the gluteal fold.

107

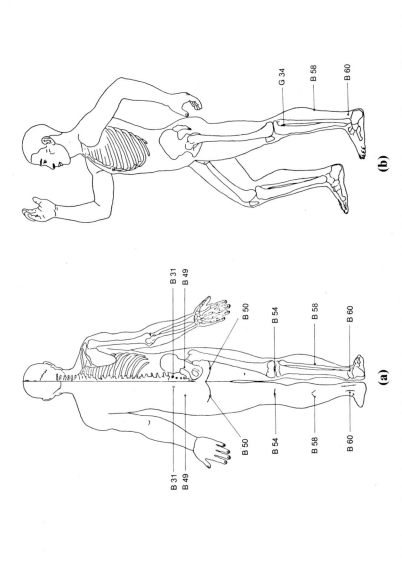

(b)

(a)

Fig. 88: Sciatica, Typical Course, Dorsal. B 31, 49, 50, 54, 58, 60; G 34 – **(a)** – B 31 = in the first sacral foramen, B 49 = 4 fingerbreadths lateral to the 4th sacral foramen (B 34), B 50 = in the middle of the gluteal fold, B 54 = in the middle of the popliteal space, B 58 = on the outer side of the calf, B 60 = midway between the external malleolus and the Achilles tendon – **(b)** – G 34 = in front of and below the capitulum of the fibula.

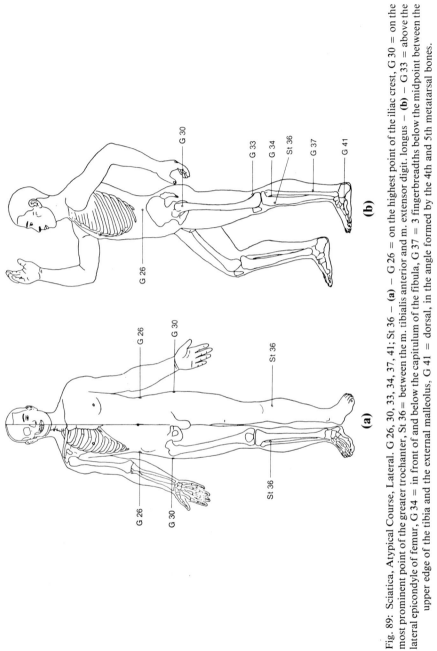

(a)

(b)

Fig. 89: Sciatica, Atypical Course, Lateral. G 26, 30, 33, 34, 37, 41; St 36 – **(a)** – G 26 = on the most prominent point of the greater trochanter, St 36 = between the m. tibialis anterior and m. extensor digit. longus – **(b)** – G 33 = above the lateral epicondyle of femur, G 34 = in front of and below the capitulum of the fibula, G 37 = 3 fingerbreadths below the midpoint between the upper edge of the tibia and the external malleolus, G 41 = dorsal, in the angle formed by the 4th and 5th metatarsal bones.

109

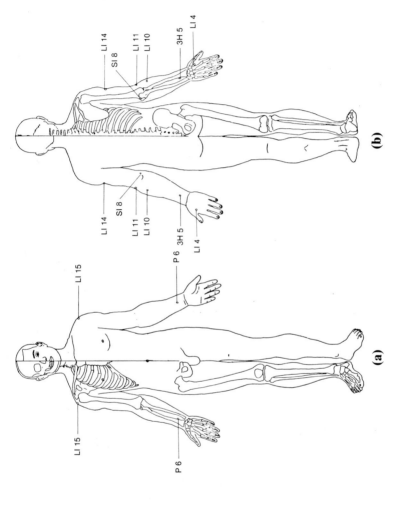

(b)

(a)

Fig. 90: Paralysis of the Upper Extremities. LI 4, 10, 11, 14, 15; SI 8, 3H 5, P 6 – **(a)** – LI 15 = on the lateral edge of the shoulder in the indentation below the acromion, P 6 = in the volar midline of the lower arm, approx. 3 fingerbreadths above the largest crease of the wrist – **(b)** – LI 14 = on the lowest point of attachment of the deltoid m., SI 8 = on the lower portion of the edge of the olecranon, LI 11 = on the lateral end of the crease of the elbow, LI 10 = approx. 2 fingerbreadths below LI 11, 3H 5 = on the dorsal midline of the lower arm, approx. 3 finger-breadths above the largest crease of the wrist, LI 4 = in the angle between the 1st and 2nd metacarpal bones.

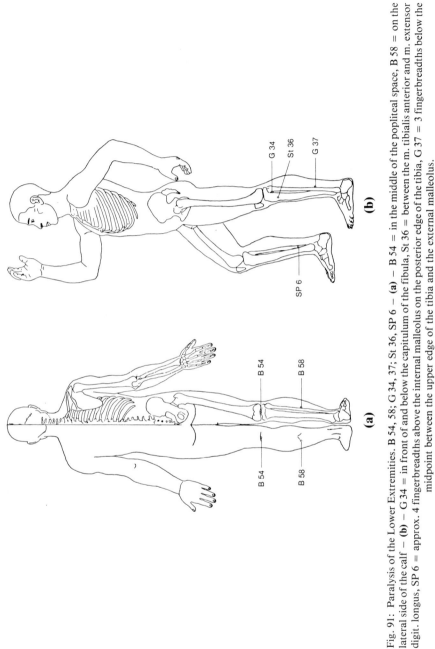

(b)

G 34
St 36
G 37

SP 6

(a)

B 54
B 58

B 54
B 58

Fig. 91: Paralysis of the Lower Extremities. B 54, 58; G 34, 37; St 36, SP 6 – **(a)** – B 54 = in the middle of the popliteal space, B 58 = on the lateral side of the calf – **(b)** – G 34 = in front of and below the capitulum of the fibula, St 36 = between the m. tibialis anterior and m. extensor digit. longus, SP 6 = approx. 4 fingerbreadths above the internal malleolus on the posterior edge of the tibia, G 37 = 3 fingerbreadths below the midpoint between the upper edge of the tibia and the external malleolus.

111

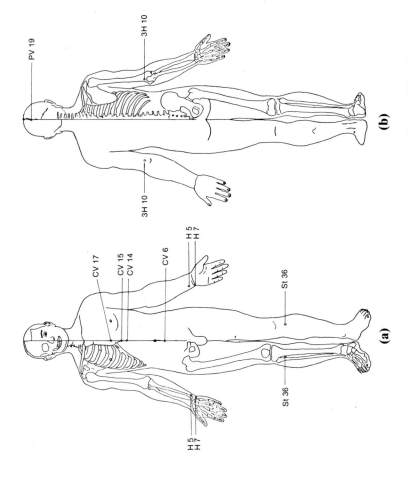

(a)

(b)

Fig. 92: Anticipatory Anxiety. CV 6, 14, 15, 17; PV 19, 3H 10, H 5, 7; St 36 – **(a)** – CV 17 = in the middle of the sternum, on the level of the 4th intercostal space, CV 15 = below the tip of the xiphoid, CV 14 = one eighth below the tip of the xiphoid, CV 6 = 2 fingerbreadths below the navel, H 5 = on the level of the ulnar apophysis, H 7 = on the radial side of the pisiform bone, St 36 = between the m. tibialis anterior and m. extensor digit. longus – **(b)** – 3H 10 = on the proximal edge of the olecranon, PV 19 = on the point of intersection of the lambdoid and sagittal sutures.

112

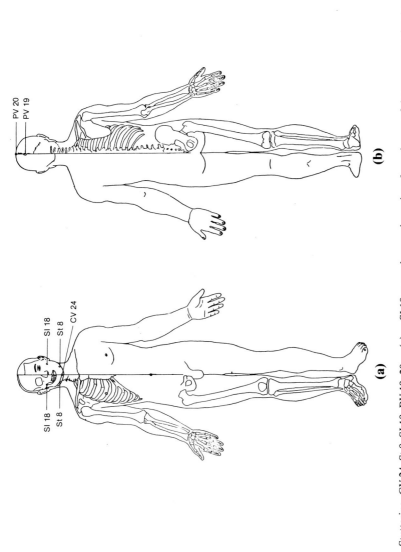

(b)

(a)

Fig. 93: Stuttering. CV 24, St 8, SI 18, PV 19, 20 – **(a)** – SI 18 = on the anterior point of attachment of the masseter to the cheek bone in the angle these form, St 8 = on the point of intersection of an imaginary perpendicular line through the middle of the pupil and the lower edge of the mandible, CV 24 = exactly on the tip of the chin – **(b)** – PV 20 = on the midline, on the highest point of the crown, PV 19 = on the point of intersection of the lambdoid and sagittal sutures.

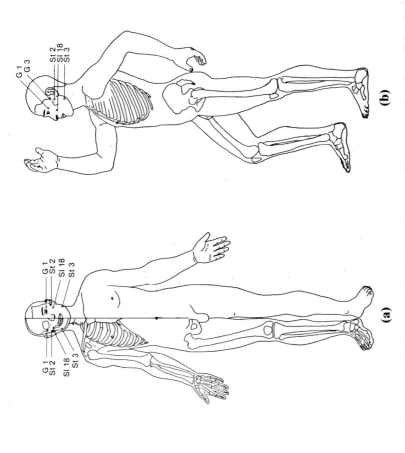

Fig. 94: Lockjaw. SI 18, G 1, 3; St 2, 3; local point – **(a)** – G 1 = in the angle orbital curve – cheek bone, St 2 = in the middle of the point of attachment of the masseter to the cheek bone, SI 18 = on the anterior point of attachment of the masseter to the cheek bone in the angle these form, St 3 = on the attachment of the masseter on the upper edge of the mandible, usually in the angle of the jaw – **(b)** – G 3 = just above the middle of the cheek bone.

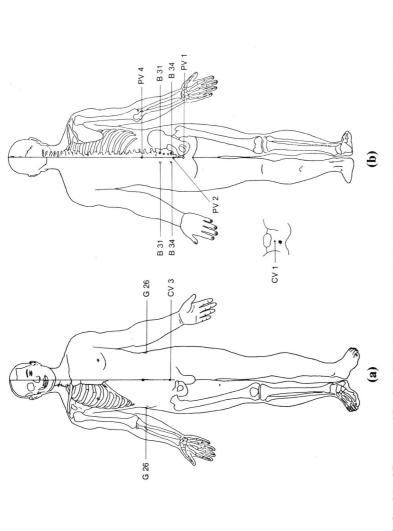

(a)

(b)

Fig. 95: Genital and Anal Eczema and Pruritus. PV 1, 2, 4; CV 1, 3; B 31, 34; G 26 – **(a)** – G 26 = on the highest point of the iliac crest, CV 3 = 2 fingerbreadths above the symphysis – **(b)** – PV 4 = on the spinous process of L 3, B 31 = in the first sacral foramen, B 34 = in the 4th sacral foramen, PV 1 = immediately behind and proximal to the anus, PV 2 = on the dorsal midline between the coccyx and sacrum. CV 1 = immediately in front of and above the anus.

115

116

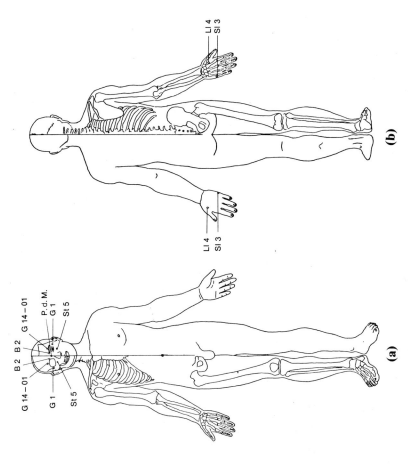

Fig. 96: Hordeolum, Conjunctivitis. LI 4, SI 3, P. d. M., B 2, St 5, G 1, 14-01 – **(a)** – B 2 = on the medial end of the eyebrow, G 14-01 = in the middle of the eyebrow, P. d. M. = in the middle of the root of the nose, G 1 = in the angle orbital curve – cheek bone, St 5 = in the infraorbital foramen – **(b)** – LI 4 = in the angle between the 1st and 2nd metacarpal bones, SI 3 = on the lateral end of the skin fold behind (proximal to) the metacarpophalangeal joint of the small finger, when the hand is closed in a fist.

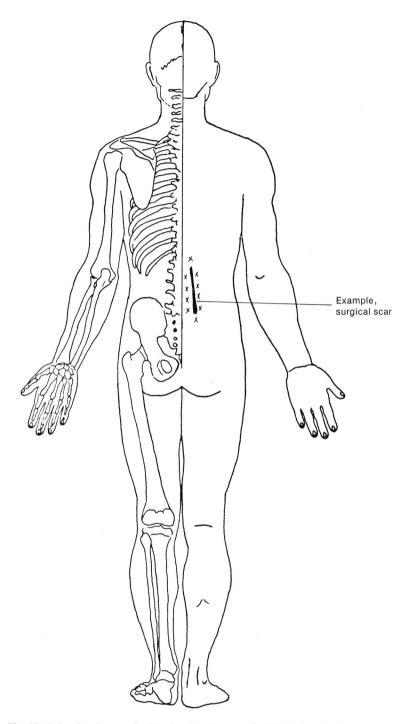

Example,
surgical scar

Fig. 97: Pain after Surgery for Hernia of an Intervertebral Disk. Local points = x.

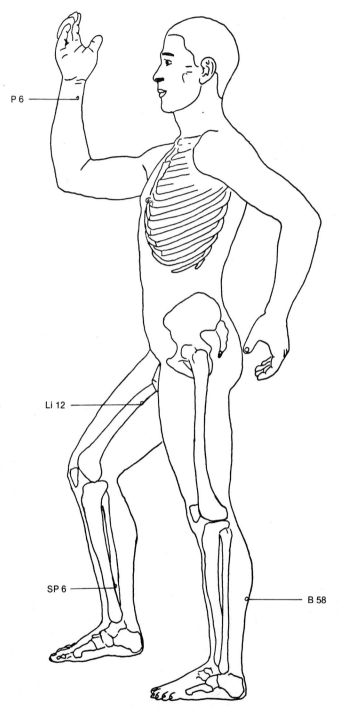

Fig. 98: Blood Supply, general. P 6, SP 6, Li 12, B 58 — P 6 = on the volar midline of the lower arm, approx. 3 fingerbreadths above the largest crease of the wrist, Li 12 = on the lower end of Scarpa's triangle, SP 6 = approx. 4 fingerbreadths above the internal malleolus, B 58 = on the outer side of the calf.

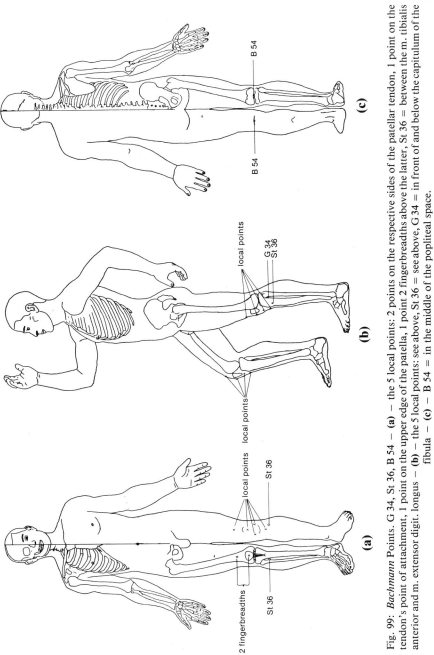

(a)

2 fingerbreadths

St 36

local points

St 36

(b)

local points

local points

local points

G 34
St 36

(c)

B 54

B 54

Fig. 99: *Bachmann* Points. G 34, St 36, B 54 – **(a)** – the 5 local points: 2 points on the respective sides of the patellar tendon, 1 point on the tendon's point of attachment, 1 point on the upper edge of the patella, 1 point 2 fingerbreadths above the latter, St 36 = between the m. tibialis anterior and m. extensor digit. longus – **(b)** – the 5 local points: see above, St 36 = see above, G 34 = in front of and below the capitulum of the fibula – **(c)** – B 54 = in the middle of the popliteal space.

119

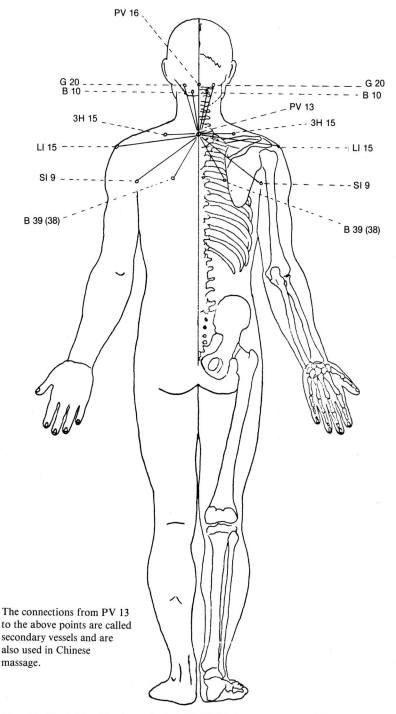

The connections from PV 13 to the above points are called secondary vessels and are also used in Chinese massage.

Fig. 100: The Spider. PV 13, 16; B 10, G 20, 3H 15, LI 15, SI 9, B 39 − PV 13 = on C 7, PV 16 = on the midline, on the lower occipital border, G 20 = on the lower occipital border, just behind the mastoid, B 10 = on the lower edge of the squama occipitalis, 2 fingerbreadths lateral to the dorsal midline, 3H 15 = on the upper edge of the trapezius in the middle of the shoulder, LI 15 = on the lateral edge of the shoulder, in the indentation below the acromion, SI 9 = 2 fingerbreadths above the dorsal end of the axillary fold, B 39 = on the point of intersection of the scapula and the upper edge of the 4th rib.

Part II

Alphabetical Index of the Control Loops

Part III

International Nomenclature of the 14 Main Channels

International Nomenclature	Nomenclature after BISCHKO	Points Cited Herein
I. P (Pulmo)	Lu (Lung)	1, 2, 5, 7, 11
II. IC (Intestinum crassum)	LI (Large Intestine)	2, 3, 4, 10, 11, 14, 15, 19, 20
III. G (Gaster)	St (Stomach)	2, 3, 5, 6, 7, 8, 9, 10, 13, 21, 25, 36, 40, 41, 42, 44, 45
IV. LP (Lien)	SP (Spleen-Pancreas)	4, 5, 6, 9
V. C (Cor)	H (Heart)	2, 3, 4, 5, 7, 9
VI. IT (Intestinum tenue)	SI (Small Intestine)	3, 4, 5, 8, 9, 18
VII. VU (Vesica urinaria)	B (Bladder)	1, 2, 4, 10, 13, 14, 15, 17, 18, 19, 20, 21, 22, 23, 25, 27, 34, 39, 47, 50, 54, 58, 60, 62, 64, 65, 67
VIII. R (Ren)	K (Kidney)	2, 6, 8, 11, 21, 27
IX. PC (Pericardium)	P (Pericardium)	6, 7, 9
X. T (Tricalori)	3H (Triple Heater)	4, 5, 10, 15, 17, 22, 23
XI. VF (Vesica fellea)	G (Gallbladder)	1, 2, 3, 8, 14, 17, 20, 26, 27, 28, 30, 33, 34, 37, 38, 40, 41, 43
XII. H (Hepar)	Li (Liver)	2, 3, 6, 8, 12, 13
XIII. TM (Toumo)	PV (Pilot Vessel)	1, 3, 4, 13, 16, 19, 20, 23
XIV. JM (Jennmo)	CV (Conception Vessel)	3, 4, 6, 9, 12, 13, 14, 15, 17, 21, 22, 24

Example of synonymous terms:

LI 4 = IC 4 = II/4
PV 13 = TM 13 = XII/13
H 7 = C 7 = V/7

Part IV

The Specific Types of Acupuncture Points

	Symbol	Type	Points
1.	●	Tonification Points:	Lu 9, SP 2, H 9, K 7, P 9, Li 8(9). LI 11, St 41, SI 3, B 67, 3H 3, G 43.
2.	∅	Sedation Points:	Lu 5, SP 5, H 7, K 1, 2; P 7, Li 2. LI 2, 3; St 45, SI 8, B 65, 3H 10, G 38.
3.	⬤	Lo Points (Passage Points):	Lu 7, LI 6, St 40, SP 4, H 5, SI 7, B 58, K 4, P 6, 3H 5, G 37, Li 5.
4.	∅	Source Points:	Lu 9, LI 4, St 42, SP 3, H 7, SI 4, B 64, K 3, P 7, 3H 4, G 40, Li 3.
5.	▲	Cardinal Points:	SP 4, G 41, P 6, 3H 5, B 62, K 6, SI 3, Lu 7.

6. ■ Associated* Points and Alarm Points:

Organ	Associated Point	Alarm Point
Lung	B 13 (Th 3)	Lu 1
Liver	B 18 (Th 9)	Li 14
Gallbladder	B 19 (Th 10)	G 24
Spleen-Pancreas	B 20 (Th 11)	Li 13
Kidney	B 23 (L 2)	G 25
Large Intestine	B 25 (L 4)	St 25
Pericardium	B 14 (Th 4)	CV 17
Heart	B 15 (Th 5)	CV 14
Stomach	B 21 (Th 12)	CV 12
Triple Heater	B 22 (L 1)	CV 5
Small Intestine	B 27 (S 1)	CV 4
Bladder	B 28 (S 2)	CV 3

		Type	Points
7.		Metabolic Points:	LI 2, LI 3, LI 4, Li 13, K 6, K 2, B 54, B 58.

---

* (or Concurring or "Assentiment")

8.   Master Points: Lu 7 (for any process in the thorax)
Lu 9 (vascular disorders, arrhythmia)
LI 3, 4 (acne)
Lu 11 (throat disorders)
LI 1 (toothache)
LI 11 (paresis of the upper extremity)
St 36 (hyper and hypotension, hormone
balance, gastro-intestinal tract)
SP 4 (any type of diarrhea)
SP 9 (female genital organs, miction)
H 3 (depression)
SI 3, Li 2, 3 (spasms, mucous
membrane)
B 31 (menopause)
B 38 (39) (hematopoiesis)
B 54 (skin diseases)
B 60 (any type of pain)
B 62, K 6 (insomnia)
P 7 (intercostal neuralgia, hypertension)
3H 4 (vascular cephalaea)
3H 5 (rheumatism)
3H 15 (sensitivity to weather)
G 30 (sciatica and paresis of the lower
extremities)
G 34 (musculature)
G 41 (pain in large joints)
PV 4 (sexual point)
PV 13 (exhaustion)
PV 19 (mental exhaustion, poor
concentration)
CV 15 (vital centers, together with
PV 19 as the "Bellergal® (belladonna)
of Acupuncture"

Part V

**The Energetic and Topographic Relationships
of the 12 Meridians**

The Energetic and Topographic Relationships of the 12 Meridians

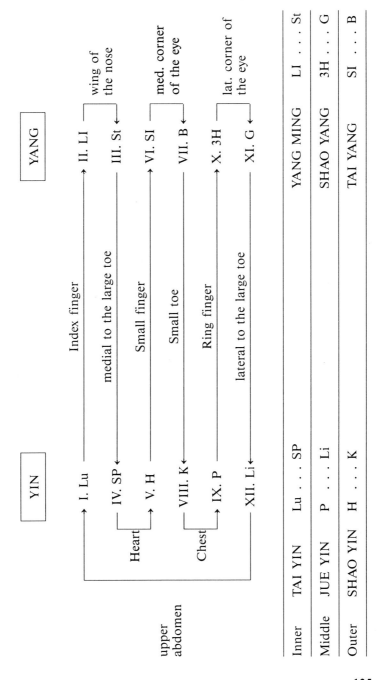

Inner	TAI YIN	Lu . . . SP	YANG MING	LI . . . St
Middle	JUE YIN	P . . . Li	SHAO YANG	3H . . . G
Outer	SHAO YIN	H . . . K	TAI YANG	SI . . . B

The Energetic and Topographic Relationships of the 12 Meridians

This is an important part of traditional Chinese medicine. The Table shows the essentials at a glance.

On the left side of the diagram, the 6 Yin organs are listed (Lu, SP, H, K, P, and Li); on the right, the 6 Yang organs (LI, St, SI, B, 3H, G).

If you follow the arrow (starting with the Meridian of the Lung), you will obtain a clear picture of the local transitions from one meridian to the next. The horizontal lines indicate meridian partners (e. g. Lu → LI, B → K).

The data underneath indicate the respective meridian courses on the upper and lower extremities. The term "inner (Tai Yin)" means radial on the upper extremity, and the corresponding course on the lower extremity (Yang Ming). Likewise, "outer (Shao Yin)" means ulnar on the upper extremity, and the corresponding course on the lower (Tai Yang). In-between these two basic lines is the "middle" (Yue Yin = upper extremity, Shao Yang = lower extremity), corresponding on the volar side of the lower arm approximately to the n. medianus.

These terms do not apply to the entire courses of the meridians, especially not on the lower extremities, but they do apply to important sections thereof, particularly on the distal parts of the extremities.

136